Senior Nurse Mentor

SENIOR NURSE MENTOR

CURING WHAT AILS
HOSPITAL NURSING MORALE

How very little can be done under a spirit of fear.
— *Florence Nightingale*

Michael W. Perry

INKLING BOOKS   AUBURN   2015

DESCRIPTION

Many nurses are unhappy. The demands on them are great and praise is rare. Conflicts between nurses are so common, there's a term for it—"Nurses eating their own." Morale is often low, turnover is high, and costly mistakes are made. Based on experiences at one of the country's top children's hospital, this book offers a practical answer, a bold new nursing specialty uniquely empowered and tasked with maintaining nursing morale. She is a senior nurse mentor and this is her story.

DEDICATION

To all the nurses who, when I knew so little, were kind enough to mentor me.

LIBRARY CATALOGING DATA

Title: *Senior Nurse Mentor: Curing What Ails Hospital Nursing Morale*
Author: Michael W. Perry (1948–).

DESCRIPTION:

130 pages and 23 pictures. Photos from Big Stock Photos and Deposit Photos used with permission.
Size: 6 x 9 x 0.3 inches, 229 x 152 x 7 mm. Weight: 0.4 pounds, 186 grams.
Library of Congress Control Number: 2015908531 (trade paperback).

BISAC SUBJECT HEADINGS

MED058110 Medical / Nursing / Management & Leadership
MED043000 Medical / Hospital Administration & Care
MED058090 Medical / Nursing / Issues

ISBN ASSIGNMENTS

Trade paperback: 978-1-58742-086-3
Epub reflowable: 978-1-58742-087-0 (iBookstore)
Epub fixed-layout: 978-1-58742-088-7 (iBookstore)
Kindle reflowable: 978-1-58742-089-4 (Amazon)
Kindle fixed layout: 978-1-58742-090-0 (Amazon)
Smashwords: 978-1-58742-091-7 (additional digital editions):

PUBLISHER INFORMATION

Print edition published in the United States of America on acid-free paper.
First edition. First printing, June 2015
Publisher: Inkling Books, Auburn, AL 36830
Internet: http://www.InklingBooks.com/

Contents

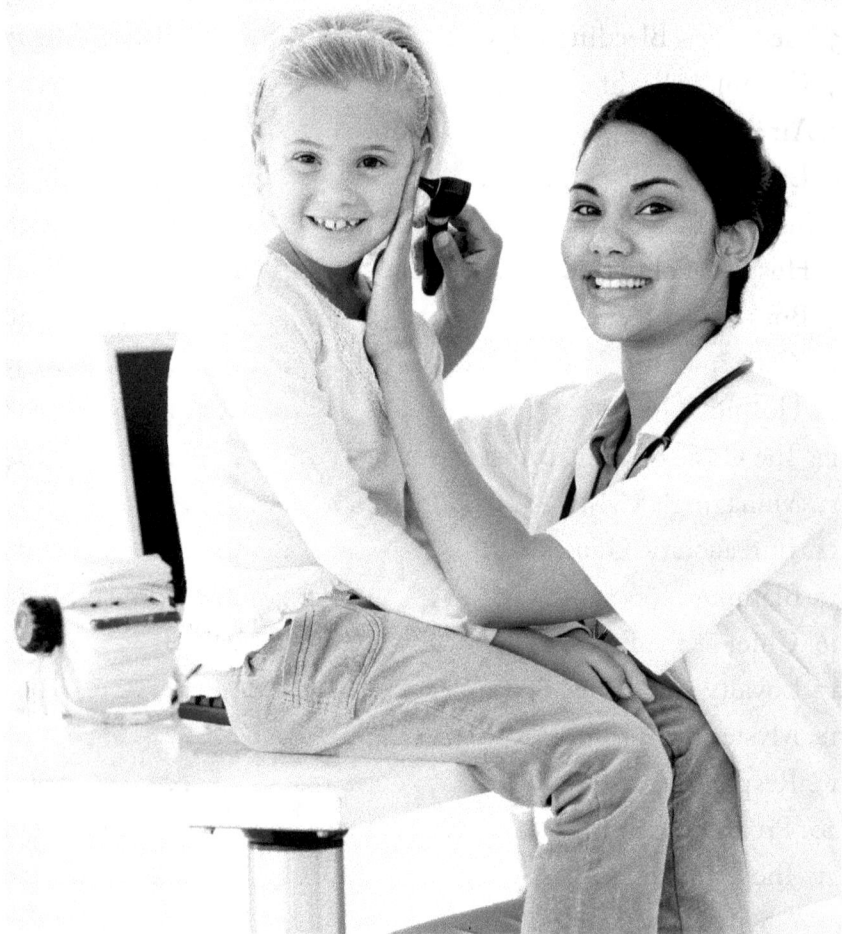

1. Why Read This?

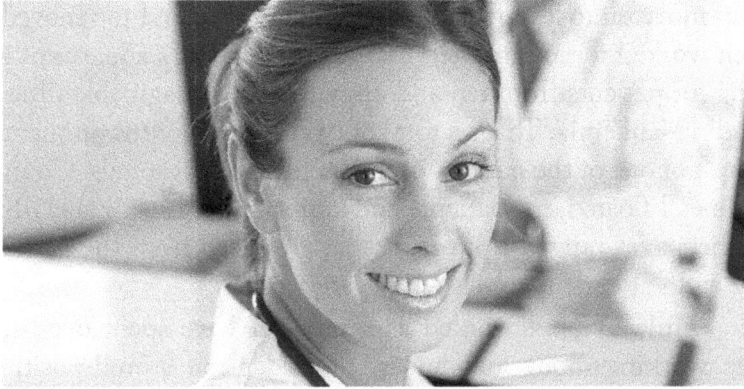

Why should you read this book? Simple, because it offers a practical solution to a problem that vexes hospital nurses—a difficult and frustrating work environment that weakens morale, harms patients, and increases medical costs. What's suggested can make life better for all involved, nurses, patients and administrators.

Why me? After all, I'm not a nurse. My formal medical training isn't in nursing. It consists of mountaineering first aid courses, Emergency Medical Technician (EMT) training at a community college, and graduate work in medical ethics in the University of Washington's medical school. I like to call the last, "studying law in a medical school."

No, that didn't make me a lawyer—thank goodness. I did, however, learn enough law to win a copyright dispute in federal court against one of the largest literary estates on the planet. When push comes to shove, I know how to fight and win. But the good news is that the answer this book offers isn't just for nurses who are as tough as nails. What it suggests will work for everyone, including those like shy young nurse pictured on the back cover of the print edition. That matters quite a bit.

Of course, that's not the whole story. I parlayed that EMT training into a nurse tech position (then called a pediatric aide) at one of the country's top-ten children's hospitals. There I worked nights alongside a nurse in the hospital's specialized Hem-Onc unit. My patients ranged from three months until their tenth birthday. Most had leukemia, so I know what it's like to work under stress.

I worked Hem-Onc for sixteen months, seeing three sets of nurses move on to less grueling assignments, before I too moved on. I then worked for another ten months on hospital's adolescent unit, caring for patients from ten and up with every imaginable illnesses, including leukemia. That's a total of twenty-six months on the nursing staff of one of the nation's premier children's hospitals. Counting the times I floated, my patients had almost every imaginable illness, and their ages ranged from babies just released from the NICU to those in their early twenties with cystic fibrosis.

So, while I've not worked as a nurse, I have spent over 4,000 hours working alongside nurses. Consider me a well-positioned observer of nursing—close enough to understand but distant enough to bring a new and unique point of view.

That's what I will offer—a refreshing look at how nursing might benefit from a new type of nurse. What I say will almost certainly delight many younger nurses who understand their need for an experienced mentor to get them through the rough spots. It'll also appeal to older nurses who've been asking themselves "What should I do next?" **Nursing needs a career path that doesn't turn talented nurses with excellent people skills into dissatisfied paper pushers. This is that path.**

Even administrators who question change will realize that the best way to deal with nursing morale is to have someone who takes that on as her main responsibility. Administering and morale-building are often like oil and water. It's hard to do both well. Delegating the latter will make an administrator's job easier.

The idea also makes financial sense. Given the close connection between nursing morale and errors, hospitals will find this money well spent. In today's nasty legal environment, avoiding but one mistake and the resulting lawsuit could save millions. In return, that will drive down the cost of malpractice insurance.

In an earlier book, *Hospital Gowns and Other Embarrassments*, I offered suggestions about how patients, particularly teen girls, could make their hospital stay less embarrassing. One reviewer raised a legitimate question. Most of my suggestions, she wrote, depend on a teen girl having enough confidence to make demands in an intimidating hospital environment. Many aren't that assertive.

In the book, I did what I could to deal with that. I offered suggestions to those girls about how to charm nurses, so they'll be delighted to make your stay better. I assured those girls that no hospital was going to deny them treatment much less discharge them because they take a stand. Good nursing, I explained, is about adapting treatment to individuals.

But in the end, that reviewer was right. All the burden should not rest on patients to speak up. Hospitals need to realize that for some patients embarrassment is even more upsetting than pain, particularly for teens. Hospitals take pain seriously. They should do the same for embarrassment.

There are numerous books that take my *Hospital Gowns* approach to the hassles that nurses suffer, particularly from their fellow nurses or a hospital administration. They give excellent advice, but they *must* assume a nurse is assertive enough to speak up. Unfortunately, not all nurses are like that. It's often the most sensitive—and thus the most in need of help—who're least able to speak out.

That's why this book belongs alongside the others. It recognizes that nurses vary in assertiveness and creates a new nursing specialty to make sure that every nurse, however shy and sensitive, gets the support she deserves. One of the saddest aspects of nursing today are the students who graduate idealist and hopeful, fall into a particularly toxic work environment, and either burn out and leave nursing altogether or become cynical and unhappy for the rest of their careers. This deals with that problem.

Now I must give this new position a name. While I have adapted an oft-used term for that new nursing specialty—nurse mentor—keep in mind I'm referring to someone with far more powers and responsibilities. That's why I refer to her as a *senior nurse mentor.*

You see an illustration of her, smiling and confident, on the front cover of this book. Hers is a position that can only be achieved after years of nursing experience and one that will require dedication. At the same time it will offer an exceptional sense of accomplishment. She will have a positive impact on the lives of an entire generation of nurses and patients.

Now back to what I did on the nursing staff, so you'll understand me better. Keep in mind that on night shift the nurse/assistant line blurred dramatically. When the nurse went on break, Hem-Onc with its critically ill children was all mine.

Even more significant, a lengthy staffing crisis I describe later meant that for almost a month a nursing student and I bore the ultimate responsibility for caring for Hem-Onc's seven vulnerable children. Like it or not—and I didn't—I became a critical-care nurse with only that paltry EMT training. Yes, that was scary. Preventing situations like that is precisely why I'm writing this book. People should not be placed in a position that far removed from their training and skills.

Although I wasn't that aware of its importance at the time, I was also a first-hand witness to two dramatic transformations in the care of children with cancer. Bone marrow transplants (BMT) had taken place as far back as the 1950s, but they were rare, experimental, and held no chance of success. At that time, childhood leukemia was a death sentence. At one East Coast hospital, 90 percent of the children admitted with leukemia died within six weeks, bleeding in every imaginable way. In the face of horrors that great, almost any treatment, however doubtful, could be justified.

By the early 1980s, that had changed dramatically. In cooperation with a world-class cancer treatment center nearby, our unit did some of the first BMTs on children that were genuine treatments rather than futile experiments. The procedure was so new, when I told a friend who worked in radiation therapy that my latest patent, a fourteen-year-old boy, had received 600 REMs of whole-body radiation, she turned to me with a shocked expression and said, "That's a lethal dose."

So it was, I replied. I then explained why a bone marrow transplant began with a radiation dose that would kill within a few weeks if the transplant did not take. A few years later, I wouldn't need to explain that. She would know. Bone marrow transplants were that new.

I also a witnessed another transformation with a far broader impact. Our children needed IVs for their chemotherapy, antibiotics, and other treatments. Every two or three days, the needle would slip out of their soft little veins and fluid would infiltrate into tissue. The child would complain to a parent about pain. The call light would go on, and either the nurse or I would discover the bad news.

Soon afterward, that child would be screaming as yet another IV had to be started. I'd hold, while the nurse did the poke. We hated it. Given everything else that the child was going through, it was a rotten, terrible, miserable, vile procedure. Still worse, after several weeks of hospitalization, we often ran out of places to poke. What we was did good medicine, but it felt more like torture.

Often there was a discussion about whether starting another IV made sense. If a child was getting medications, it was. But what if he or she wasn't? Our kids had endured so much, did we have to start another IV just in case? While the decision was the responsibility of the resident on duty that night, nursing experience usually trumped rank. In the middle of the night, the nurse and I usually decided, and the resident followed. It wasn't a pleasant decision.

Thankfully, I soon saw that horror fade. Central lines changed everything. As with those bone marrow transplants, we were the pioneers. One of our physicians had invented a still-popular central line about two years earlier. It used a soft Silastic (rubbery) tube inserted into the upper-right chest and placed into a major vein just before it returned to the heart. When our nurses complained that the line didn't spare a child the misery of daily pokes for blood samples, this kindest of physicians modified it so it could be used to draw blood as well as give fluids. For us—and especially for those children—that was utterly wonderful.

When I started, central lines were the exception. Within a few months they were the rule. After diagnosis and workup, cancer treatment would begin with the insertion of a central line. Properly cared for, that line could stay in place for months, sparing a child numerous pokes. Caring for that line and doing the daily blood draw became a part of the regular routine for night shift.

Unfortunately, the leading edge of technology is also the bleeding edge. That's when the worst mistakes are made. For our Hem-Onc specialists, the learning curve centered on those early bone marrow transplants. Two of the boys I cared for who received BMTs died. One died of an infection that fell into a narrow gap between two broad-spectrum antibiotics. The other died of graft-versus-host disease (GVH) despite the fact that the donation came from his twin brother.

This book stresses lessons that flow from that other learning curve, the one connected with those then-new central lines and the risks associated with them. That experience and the accompanying mistakes—which quickly spread with the central lines from Hem-Onc to the entire hospital—may have contributed to a final climatic experience I'll discuss, a clash between the hospital administration and its nurses so intense, some twenty percent of the nurses quit and replacing them became almost impossible.

Seeing that situation develop, step by terrible step, is the key reason why I have the expertise to write this book. I have seen all too vividly how a hospital's nursing morale can collapse, little by little, over the space of some two years. If you want a rough parallel, imagine a naval conference on great passenger vessel disasters. I'd be the speaker who'd been an officer on the *Titanic*. I know what disaster looks like and it isn't pretty.

Those experiences provide a foundation for a new nursing position, a senior nurse mentor who is *independent* of most administrative controls and *tasked* with playing a critical role in nurse training and morale. She and the possibilities that she offers are why this book is worth reading. My experiences merely provide the backdrop. She's the one you should be thinking about.

The day might even come when you become one.

2. My Nights with Leukemia

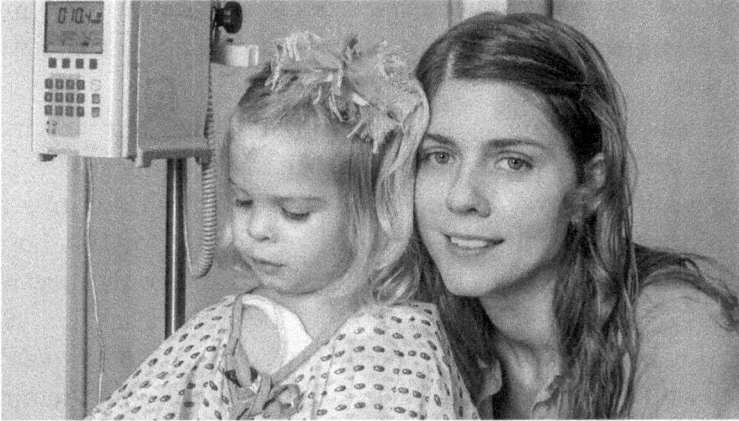

Ican't begin a book about nurses as mentors without mentioning the wonderful nurses who mentored me when I needed it most—when I first began to work on Hem-Onc with only the woefully inadequate 'scoop and run' training of a medic.

That story begins with an odd twist. Mountain climbing in the Pacific Northwest taught me the importance of knowing emergency medicine. Anything could happen in the mountains far from assistance. As a result, I took Emergency Medical Technician (EMT) training at a community college. I thought about becoming a medic-volunteer with a mountain search and rescue team.

Then my life took dramatic U-turn. Headed for bankruptcy, the energy management firm where I worked laid me off. A friend suggested I apply for a nursing assistant job at a nearby children's hospital. I was accepted for a position on the medical unit's night shift that would start after a month of orientation on days.

I soon wondered if I'd made the right choice. Day shift meant endless busy work that I found dull. I'm simply not cut out for linen changes and the like. I like challenge. But I hung in there, hoping night shift would prove different.

I also knew what I did not want to do on nights. There was one challenge I did not want. I did not want to work on Hem-Onc. The hospital is different now, with two independent units dedicated to childhood and adolescent cancers. But at that time children up to their tenth birthday were handled on one cluster (seven beds) of the three-cluster, children-from-one-to-nine medical unit where I was assigned. Elsewhere in the hospital, teens with cancer were mixed with the general population of the adolescent unit. Later I would work there.

Why didn't I want to work Hem-Onc? I explain why in *My Nights with Leukemia*. Here, I'll just state that looking at Hem-Onc from mere yards away horrified me. The children being treated—most of them had leukemia—looked like the survivors of a horrible concentration camp. They were thin and pale, with only a few wisps of hair. I breathed a sigh of relief when I looked over at them, stumbling slowly alongside a parent who was pushing an IV pole festooned with bags and pumps. Hem-Onc was nurse-only, I reminded myself. I would never work there.

Then my orientation ended. I appeared for my first night shift and discovered that I was assigned to Hem-Onc. Night shift wasn't all-RN. It paired a nurse with and an assistant. I was to be that assistant. Later, the hospital's director of nursing would tell me that my EMT training had given me what was probably the most demanding assistant position in the hospital. To staff it seven days a week, it had two assistant slots. I shared my position with someone I will call Cala, a student at a top-notch nursing school nearby.

Fortunately, my situation rapidly turned from fearful to positive. I discovered that I loved carrying for those children and came to believe I had a knack for the many stresses and emotional complications. I had found my niche at that hospital.

Alas, Cala loved the work as much as I did, and several nights out of every fourteen we were both on duty. We clashed until we reached an agreement. Whoever had been working Hem-Onc would continue to do so when the other returned from break. That gave those children continuity. When I came back, she continued to care for them. Several days later, when she left, I'd learned enough from her to take over and vice-versa.

There was another hitch, an enormous one for me. Cala was in her third year of school and thus almost a nurse. I only had a couple of mountaineering first aid courses and that EMT training—three hours on three nights a week for three months. That was roughly a hundred hours in emergency medicine. I knew how to stop serious external bleeding, temporarily splint broken bones, and deliver untimely babies. I'd been taught nothing about childhood leukemia.

Fortunately, I arrived at the perfect time. Three experienced nurses took turns filling the Hem-Onc night-nurse position. That's when my mentoring began. As I explain in *My Nights*, they taught me well. At the time, I didn't appreciate just how vital their mentoring would be. Children's lives would soon depend on what I had learned from them about good nursing.

Here's what that work was like. On days, two Hem-Onc nurses divided up the patients, with one nurse caring for four children and the other for three. On nights, the division was based on the work done. The nurses complained that night shift meant carrying for IV pumps rather than children. They were right. Seven children meant seven complex IV systems to manage—that I'll discuss in more detail later. Treatment went on around the clock, so night shift got its full share of IV care. As a result, night shift meant a nurse was constantly moving between IVs, wrapping up chemotherapy with one child while giving antibiotics to another.

That left the hands-on patient care to Cala and I. We were the ones who checked vital signs, looking especially for a temperature spike that meant infection. We made sure that, with so much fluid being pumped into a child, their urine output remained high. There was also time to built friendships with the children during those scary nights when we took over so parents could get much-needed sleep. Caring for the same children for weeks at a time and getting to know them was why Cala and I loved what we were doing.

A humorous incident a couple of months after I started illustrates how well they had trained me. One of those first nurses was giddily happy married to an officer on a Coast Guard cutter, and he had just come back from a six-week cruise. She was spending so much time with him, she arrived at work one evening almost falling asleep.

After she'd completed her 4 a.m medications, she told me she'd be napping during her break, a half-hour in the middle of the night that substituted for the usual lunch or dinner break. I thought nothing of it. The kids were stable, and if a crisis came up, I could always call on the nurse on the next cluster. I didn't notice that she hadn't told me to wake her.

Doing her work and mine kept me so busy that I wasn't aware of the passing time until the head nurse arrived almost two hours later. "Not good," I thought. "She didn't intend to sleep this long." As unobtrusively as possible, I slipped over to the next cluster and asked its nurse to cover any alarms on Hem-Onc.

Then I began searching for Sleeping Beauty. Fortunately, she was in the mostly likely place, a couch in the nursing locker room. I woke her and hurried back. She arrived a couple of minutes later, doing her best to conceal that she'd just awakened from a deep sleep. For once our head nurse's thick head served us well. She noticed nothing. What happens on night shift stays on night shift.

That bit of mischief illustrates how well I'd been taught. Just keep in mind that what I knew well was the routine care for one particular kind of patient. There's no substitute for years of nursing school and work as a nurse rather than an assistant.

Learning on the job like that, with little time spent in classrooms, probably couldn't happen in today's more formal job market. An informal apprenticeship had transformed me from an ambulance-trained EMT into a specialized nurse tech. In about two months I'd gone from being terrified at the prospect of working on Hem-Onc to being able to handle its routine work so calmly, I hardly noticed when I served for a couple of hours as both nurse and assistant. The work had become as natural as breathing.

However, my new-found ability would severely tested when a major crisis hit Hem-Onc shortly afterward. When it struck, Cala and I would become Hem-Onc's *de facto* nurses for several long and terrifying weeks.

That's next. Later, I will draw some important lessons from what seemed at the time to be no more than an unplanned disaster.

3. Medicine's Bleeding Edge

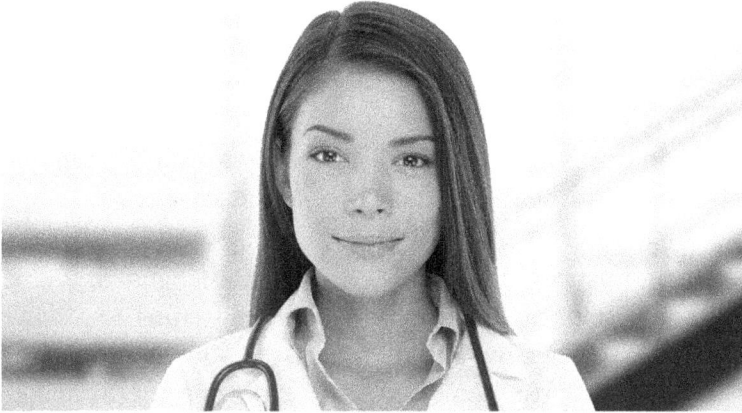

"You're grinding your teeth," my dentist said, "that's what is causing your mouth to ache." A sports mouth guard would take care of the grinding, he said. I'd have to take care of the stress myself.

I knew what was causing that stress. My first few months on Hem-Onc had been great. Three experienced nurses taught me well. New to nursing, to hospital work, and to pediatric cancer, I now knew what was expected of me. But the roots of that stress did not lie in what I was supposed to do. I could do that well. It lay in an almost impossible set of additional expectations that had suddenly been thrust on Cala and me.

For differing reasons, all three night nurses left within a few weeks, resulting in a woeful loss of expertise that would have been difficult to fill at best. What happened next was far from ideal.

First, it's hard to find experienced nurses for night shift, so the hospital hired three recent graduates. That might have worked if their orientation had been well-executed. It wasn't. The orienting nurse believed in 'toss them in and see if they sink.' They were expected to learn on their own.

That resulted in a second problem. The orienting nurse showed them a procedure once, and then told them to come to her at the nursing station if they had problems. As you might guess, those new nurses muddled through their orientation on their own, not learning all the gotchas. Even before their orientation was over, that lack of aggressive training had me worried. I'd been trained well by three nurses, each with different approaches to patient care. I didn't think these three were being trained equally well by this one nurse.

Worse of all was the third problem. Two of the three new nurses simply weren't that good. As with any field, some people have a knack for nursing, and some don't. These two didn't. One would openly admit it. The other seemed better at covering up her mistakes—something I found scary.

As their mistakes multiplied, my work changed dramatically. For over three months, at report I had been listening to a conversation between the evening and night nurses. Now the evening nurse seemed to give report to me—silently expecting me to make sure nothing went wrong. Cala faced the same pressures, but she had far more experience, along with those three years of nursing school. I had terribly little experience and almost no formal training. That's where my stress came from. I *felt* overwhelmed, because I *was* overwhelmed.

Parents reacted much like the evening nurses. Their child's long hospitalization made them good at spotting trouble. Sensing those mistakes, they began to cling to Cala and I for support. We were the only ones not making mistakes. We became their only hope. That brought still more stress. I had to reassure them even though I felt none too secure myself.

Nor could Cala and I turn to the night residents for help. One came around, at best, for a few minutes each night, and each spent only six weeks with our unit before moving on. Most had enough sense to take their lead from nursing staff. They needed us more than we needed them.

As a result, Cala and I became Hem-Onc's final line of defense. It was us or nobody. As best I could tell, she coped well. I felt like a drowning man, struggling to stay on top of the water with one notable exception. If I failed, I wouldn't die, but a child might. Only a few months before I'd hardly known what leukemia was. Now I was expected to manage the night care of seven children battling for their lives. I not only could not make any mistakes of my own, I had to catch any mistakes those new nurses might make. *There is no scary like that kind of scary.*

Fortunately, the situation could have been worse. I was already doing what mattered most. In the night-time division of labor, I was the one who watched over the kids. Yes, odd as it may sound, the most critical task on Hem-Onc was given to the assistant—those vital signs and the brief interaction with the child they brought. More than ever before, I needed to do that well, letting nothing that happened to those children escape my attention.

Drugs were not that great a worry. With the exception of narcotics, all the medications we gave came well-marked and in the proper doses from the pharmacy every four hours. Its staff were experienced, so I could depend on them. Fortunately, at that time we had no one on morphine, which came from our own locked cabinet.

That left only the IVs themselves. That's where the trouble lay, especially with our new central lines. There were several reasons why that was true.

First, the IV treatments for our children were extremely complicated. Two or even three IV pumps were the norm. From a child's IV pole hung several IV bags that often looked alike. Seven kids with two or more pumps each meant that at night a single nurse was often managing 15 or more IV pumps and even more treatments.

The difficulties didn't ease after their initial treatment. Our chemotherapy destroyed their blood, often necessitating antibiotics for infections, along with platelets and red blood cells when needed. Since these children often did not feel like eating, we gave them the empty calories of D40W or more long-term hyperalimentation (also known as Total Parenteral Nutrition or TPN), along with lipids to meet their nutritional needs. Today, much simpler NG tube feedings are common.

Each treatment came with its own set of requirements. Some fluids could not be given at the same time as others, which meant one pump needed to be stopped, changed, and restarted. Some drugs were well-understood. Others, including powerful anti-viral drugs, were experimental or dangerous and needed carefully monitoring. Even for experienced nurses, that would have been hard.

Now imagine yourself as a recent nursing school graduate. In nursing school, you took care of one, two or perhaps three patients. One of them might have an IV with but a single bag of fluids. At that time, none would have a central line with the additional complications that brought.

Most nursing students, I later discovered, made that experience even less realistic. They took care to keep their work load small, simple, and safe. When I worked days on the teen unit, out of self-interest I tried to get student nurses to take a more difficult patient. Almost all chose someone easy to care for. "Hey," I felt like telling them, "when you graduate, lives will depend on you not making mistakes. You *must* get used to difficulties now." Students pay for that caution when they become nurses and face a much heavier work load with no backup and no one they can run to for help.

Now imagine that, as a recent nursing graduate, you're responsible for seven critically ill children, almost all with complex IVs. You'd be confused, wouldn't you? These new nurses certainly were. That quick orientation did not help, particularly the lack of stress on checking and rechecking any change to an IV. For my part, I never made any change to an IV without following the fluid flow from bag to patient, making sure every detail was right. I'd been taught well.

Now toss in two more complications, both born during that recent shift from traditional peripheral IVs to those otherwise wonderful central lines. Central lines were new. Even experienced nurses were still learning how to handle them. You can imagine how difficult they might be for recent nursing graduates who'd not been taught about them, particularly the risk of an air embolism.

In fact, while researching *My Nights*, I read a book about leukemia treatment at a large East Coast children's hospital two years *after* my experience on the West Coast. It made no mention of central lines. What even some top hospitals weren't doing at that time certainly wasn't being taught in nursing schools. It was that new.

I was fortunate. The first nurses I worked with taught me about the risks of an air embolism in a central line and how to handle it. Given that the doctor who'd invented what is still today one of the most popular of those lines worked at our hospital, they may have learned directly from him. That meant that when I learned I was only one step removed from the world's leading expert on such lines. Soon, that top-notch training would become critically important.

The problem with central lines is easy to explain. A bubble of air introduced into a vein in the arm has ample time to break up and dissolve before it reaches the heart. In contrast, our central line entered a major vein in a slow-moving blood flow only a few inches from the heart. After a quick pass through the heart to the lungs and back, that bubble could be pumped out, still large and intact, to the heart or brain, perhaps shutting off a critical blood supply. That was bad, bad, bad.

That's why those first nurses taught me that when I saw air in a patient's line, I was to instantly turn off the IV pump, lower the child's head, roll the child on his or her left side and elevate the lower part of his or her body. Hopefully, that meant that those dangerous air bubbles, being more buoyant than blood, would lodge in the lungs where they would do less harm.

Are you seeing the problem? First, came those complex IVs and the confusion they created. Second came central lines and the risk of a dangerous air embolism that had to be treated quickly and correctly. Unfortunately, there was yet one more problem that, joined to the others, created a perfect storm of trouble.

Our central lines were new, but our IV pumps were several years old and not designed to be used with such lines. They had a critical failing. The sensor that detected air wasn't built into the pump itself like it is today. It had to be manually clipped to an IV line. With our complex IVs and constant fluid changes, that meant the air sensor could accidentally be placed on the wrong line. There it would sit, patiently watching for air on an unused line while the actual line pumped a stream of air into a patient. That was a terrible flaw.

Those were the risk factors. But for disaster to happen, a nurse still had to make a mistake. Next, we look at how those mistakes were made.

4. Getting It Right

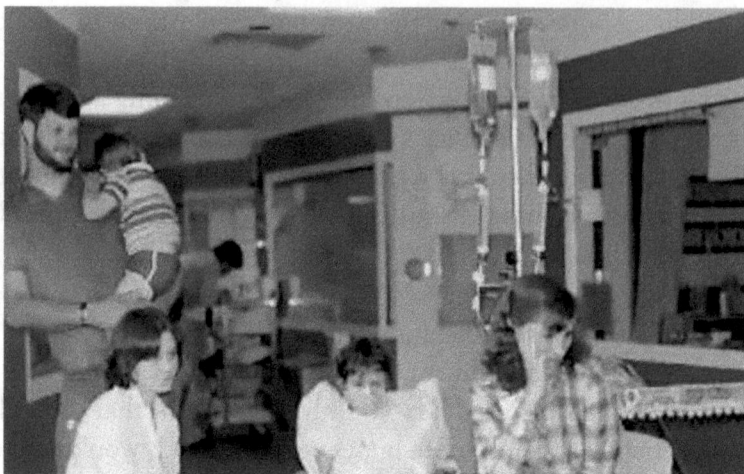

How did those risk factors for central lines become actual medical emergencies? IV setups can vary. I'll explain ours, so you'll understand where the troubles lay.

You see our typical installation in the picture above, taken at a birthday party for a patient. The boy was wearing a mask, so his white count must have been low. Two one-liter bags of fluid hang high on a pole. The one on the left was his chemotherapy, given in a 24-hour infusion, while the one on the right contained bicarbonate to keep his urine pH around 6.5. That was a major part of our induction chemotherapy.

From each bag came a clear plastic line with a roller valve to shut off the flow. Next there was a calibrated cylinder that could hold about 60 ml of fluid and below that a drip chamber. A special clear plastic line then went from the drip chamber around a rotating wheel on the IV pump (out of sight). As that wheel rotated, fluid was pumped through a line several feet long into the boy. Not shown in the picture was an air sensor clipped to each line just below the pump. Since our children usually had at least two IVs pumps (as here), close to them was a connector to merge the two lines and allow one or both to be turned on.

That was not complicated in itself. Once set up, it could run without attention for hours. There was but a single path for the fluid to take from the IV bag to the patient. Get the initial setup right, and there would be no problems. Unfortunately, our IVs were rarely that simple. With increasing complexity came a greater chance for mistakes.

There were two problem areas, each involving changes in fluid flow. The first was the most common. Many of our children got medications such as antibiotics every four hours. That meant shifting the IV from maintenance to medication mode and back again.

In maintenance mode, the roller valve from the IV bag was open and the filtered air valve on the cylinder was closed. With the cylinder air-tight, every drop of fluid pulled out by the pump was replaced by another drawn down from the IV bag. Set up that way, the IV would run as long as there was fluid in the bag.

To give a medication, the nurse would open the air valve and fill the cylinder with about 20 ml. of fluid. She'd then close the roller valve so no more fluid would enter from the IV bag. She'd leave open the air valve at the top of the cylinder, so air could come in to replace the fluid as it went out. Medicine would be injected into the cylinder through another opening and enter the patient with the fluid. The air sensor on the IV pump would alarm when that fluid ran out, and the nurse would run in another 20 ml of fluid to rinse the medication out of the cylinder and IV line. After that, she'd convert the IV back to maintenance mode until the next medication.

That seems so straight-forward, you might wonder why any nurse would get it wrong. In fact, I did the latter conversion hundreds of times during my sixteen months on the Hem-Onc unit without making a single mistake. Most nights, the only opportunity a nurse had for a break came after her 4 a.m. medications. She ran in the medications, typically for three or four kids, then started the rinse, after which she left on break, depending on me to flip those IVs from medication back to maintenance mode once the rinse finished.

When that switch was made, the only real hitch came with those two valves. Leave both closed, and the IV pump had no way to draw in air or fluid. The cylinder would crumple, which can be amusing but not dangerous. The danger came when a nurse forgot to change the valves when she went from medication to maintenance mode—leaving the air valve open and the roller valve closed. With so much to do, it was an easy mistake to make. With that mistake, when the fluid in the cylinder ran out the IV pump became an air pump. Air came in through the cylinder's air valve and was pumped toward the patient.

Fortunately, there was that air sensor. When the air in the line reached it, an alarm would sound. But that was the weakest link in an already troubled chain. If the sensor was on the wrong IV line, it would never alarm. The portability of that air sensor created the risk. Better engineering would have built the air sensor into the rotor itself, so it could never be on the wrong IV line. That's how IV pumps are built today. But like it or not, we had to work with that separate sensor. We were on the bleeding edge of a new technology.

The critical mistake came most often in the second problem area, one in which the IV line being used by a pump needed to be changed. Some children had two pumps but three or more different treatments, each with its own line and sharing time on those two pumps. An IV pump might be used with a nutrition bag ordinarily, switched to normal saline for an antibiotic, then switched back to nutrition once the antibiotic was run it. At times, we also needed to give blood products, adding still more complications.

In a hurry, in a dark room, in the middle of the night, and tasked with a complicated set of changes for as many as seven children, it was easy to forget to move that air sensor. Perhaps 20 minutes later, when what fluid was present in the cylinder cleared, that IV began to pump air rather than fluid. That's what created an air embolism.

Remember, this was a known problem before those new nurses arrived. That's why I'd been taught to recognize and deal with it. Since no nurse can be everywhere at once, I soon made a habit of flicking on the flashlight that hung around my neck and scanning a child's IV lines whenever I entered a room. I got good at that, and it only took a few seconds.

With the background explained, we return to that crisis on Hem-Onc. That already-in-place check I was making became critical with these new nurses. My stress level skyrocketed, as I worked alongside these inexperienced, badly oriented, and not-very-capable nurses. What I'd been doing as a matter of routine, now went into overdrive. I pushed myself to move quickly, making my rounds as fast as possible, constantly checking IVs and making sure nothing was wrong.

Twice, once for each of those less-capable nurses, I discovered an IV pumping air into a child. Sadly, one was a wonderfully sweet nine-year-old girl who had a stroke the next day. The nurse herself blamed the air embolism for the stroke.

The child whose embolism was caused by the other less talented nurse did not seem to suffer any bad consequences. A few weeks later, however, I was upset to discover through a chance remark that the she hadn't filed an incident report on the air embolism I'd discovered. Failures were leading to cover-ups. Not good at all.

Fortunately, enough incident reports were being filed about a host of mistakes that the administration realized night shift had serious problems. The two nurses responsible for most errors were required to undergo a second orientation. That proved enough. While I've describe them as less-capable, they weren't incompetent. After about two months, their skill level went up. The stress Cala and I were experiencing went down dramatically. I could concentrate on doing my job again.

A few months later, I got what I can only assume was a reward. Normally, I went to sleep as soon as I got home from night shift. For some reason, one day I didn't. I thought I could catch enough sleep in the afternoon and early evening. I set an alarm for about 10:30 that evening. I lived within walking distance of the hospital, so that gave me enough time to get there by 11. Instead, I slept through the alarm, only waking up about midnight, when I got a phone call from the hospital.

When I arrived a frantic fifteen minutes later, the night supervisor was criticizing the night nurses for not contacting her when I failed to show. She never offered a word of criticism to me and, for all I know my belated arrival never made its way into my personnel file. I'd helped the hospital out in a pinch. It had returned the favor.

About six months later, that second set of nurses acquired enough seniority to move to positions on days or evenings. The hospital had learned a lesson. The nurses in the third set were well above average. Two had been honor students. One was so smart, I wondered why she hadn't gone to medical school. That was a great relief.

Of course, even with that third set of nurses settled in and doing well, I continued to check those troublesome IVs when I entered a child's room. I did catch another air-in-line incident with one of the new nurses. In that case, the air was still about two feet away from the patient, so no harm was done. But that incident did point out that the hospital continued to face serious issues pairing old IV pumps with new central lines, especially for nurses juggling multiple, complex IVs. It needed to do more than it was doing, and especially it needed to train its nurses in the new technology.

That's our next topic.

5. Air in Line

After sixteen months on nights and with a third set of nurses now moving to other shifts, I was exhausted and needed change. A position opened up on the teen unit's day shift, so I took it. Fortunately, I brought my Hem-Onc skills with me. I would need them.

It was early afternoon. As I passed the room of a sixteen-year-old girl with leukemia, she began an unusual, tickle-in-the-throat cough. I'd heard it before and knew what it could mean. 'Air in line!' flashed through my mind. I darted in and checked the clear plastic tubing that ran into the central line on her upper chest. It had air rather than fluid—a dangerous and potentially lethal situation.

I knew what to do for the same reason I knew her cough might be a sign. That had happened enough times, my response was instinctive. For a dangerous situation flowing from a serious nursing error, having that much experience is not good. It illustrates just how serious the problem had become. Bad was almost routine.

At the same moment, I switched off this girl's IV pump with my right hand, pulled the pillow out from under her head with my left, and asked her to turn onto her left side. I then elevated the foot of her bed. That would keep the air bubbles away from her heart or brain, where they would do the most harm.

A few minutes later, when a resident arrived, all he added to my response was to give her oxygen to clear the nitrogen from her blood more quickly. Fortunately, all had gone well. I'd probably caught her air embolism within seconds after it started.

Here, I should make an aside. I suspect that tickle-in-the-throat symptom I described is a result of the particular kind of air embolism we were experiencing. An IV pumping air will release a tiny string of bubbles that must tickle some nerve in the throat, hence that peculiar cough.

Today's IV pumps with their built-in sensors make that problem much less likely. Reading the literature, the problem now lies in a different area. A central line that suddenly disconnects near a patient can result in a large bubble of air being drawn into the vein at once. That bubble is likely to lead to different or no signs, so staff should not depend on a cough as a warning like I did that day. Situations do change.

I felt good that I'd caught the problem and responded so quickly. But the reaction from the nurse I was working with worried me. When I told her what had happened, she said that if she had discovered that air embolism, she would not have known what to do.

We've now reached a critical point in my story. The fact that a nurse with several years of experience did not know the proper response to what was becoming a common emergency is one reason why I'm writing this book. Her situation—more common than it should have been—raises issues we must resolve.

Look at the context. During my sixteen months on Hem-Onc, the most serious *nursing* errors I saw were air embolisms involving those new central lines. The only error I saw that was more serious was one made by a *resident* when he wrote a morphine order with a power-of-ten mistake that a nurse did not catch. That little boy might have died if the parents had not been awake with the lights on at 1 a.m. when the boy stopped breathing. Ninety-nine nights out of a hundred, that would not have been the case. That was how close that boy came to dying.

In one sense, the hospital was well aware of its embolism problem and was taking steps to address it. During my last month on Hem-Onc, they began testing new IV pumps. They'd be finishing up that testing almost a year later when I left the hospital. At several thousand dollars each for the more sophisticated models, it was a major expense. The hospital was taking the problem seriously at the procurement level.

On the other hand, where was the training needed to teach nurses how to prevent, discover, and deal with air embolisms? Unfortunately, it didn't exist.

Remember, Hem-Onc was at the nation's ground zero for these wonderful new central lines with their accompanying problems. If there had been a class on the topic, I would have heard about it and eagerly attended. I knew what to do only because those first nurses as mentors had taught me.

There's a parallel that illustrates how the right response to an air embolism should be taught. Much of my mountain climbing was on Mt. Rainier, the only mountain in the lower 48 states with an extensive system of glaciers. Glaciers are formed when snow falls too high up on a mountain to melt away each summer. Instead the snow piles up, often growing to be hundreds of feet thick, and is transformed into ice. The resulting mass becomes so heavy that it slowly slides down the mountain, typically a few feet a day. Eventually, it reaches a low-enough elevation that it melts and feeds water into rivers.

The slopes of a glacier are dangerous. They're often steep enough that someone who slips will slide out of control on the icy surface, unable to stop themselves. The movement of the glacier also opens up deep cracks called crevasses into which a climber can fall. Some are visible. Others are covered with snow.

That's why climbers on glaciers rope themselves to other climbers. If one careens down the slope or falls into a crevasse, his fellow climbers can halt him. They do that by hurling themselves at the snow, driving their snow axe deep into the glacier, gripping that ice axe tightly, and arching their backs, digging into the snow with the spiked crampons on their boots. Hopefully, that will be enough to stop a falling climber. It does work. The one time I did a real-life arrest turned out to not be an emergency, but I did leave the other climber suspended in the air part of the way down the face of a small ice cliff.

To be sure of succeeding, an arrest must be done in an instant. If the arresting climber drives his ice axe into the snow *before* that rope snaps taut, the arrest is likely to go well. If he's *a split second too late*, he'll be plunging down the slope himself, making arrest difficult.

Dealing with an air embolism is equally time-critical. Done quickly, an air bubble that might have triggered a stroke or a heart attack never forms. But even a second of delay may be too late. That's why my response to that teen girl was so unhesitatingly quick.

Given the hospital's recent bad experiences, the proper response to air in a central line should have been drilled into the heads of every nurse in the hospital. They needed formal training as intense as my personal experiences had been. Responding to an air embolism must be a reflex as quick and instinctive as a mountain climber's ice axe arrest, waiting only for a trigger event.

How serious was the problem at that time? Two sets of numbers illustrate that. As I researched this book, I came across a statistic. Pennsylvania requires that hospitals report all air embolism incidents. In a recent year, the total for all the hospitals in the state was about eighty.

Compare that to my own experience. As but one member of the nursing staff working one shift on one unit at one hospital in a less populous state, I'd personally dealt with *four embolisms*. That was not just hearing about them. No, I was the one who actually spotted them. Were I in the Pennsylvania of today, I'd have been closely involved in five percent of the entire state's incidents. That's extremely unlikely. But it does indicate just how common air embolisms were at our hospital at that time, particularly with those inexperienced night nurses. As the cutting edge, we had become the terribly bleeding edge.

Look at the situation from a different angle. During my 26 months at the hospital, I was part of about four codes where patients stopped breathing. That's why the hospital recognized the importance of knowing CPR. It required every member of the staff to take a class each year, so they'd be ready. I know because I taught some of those classes.

Yet no one was teaching classes on air embolism. It wasn't that the hospital had no one to teach such a class. After all, the inventor of that central line was one of our physicians. He'd taught the nurses who'd taught me and could have trained teachers. The hospital also had nurses who specialized in caring for central lines. They could have taught those classes. In fact, if the hospital needed an air embolism instructor, I could have taught that class as easily as I taught CPR. I had a wealth of experience—far more than I wanted.

If anything, dealing with an air embolism correctly was more important than CPR. If a child stopped breathing, a nurse could hit a Code Blue button on the wall and within two minutes a highly skilled code team would arrive from the ICU to take over. In that short time, whether CPR was done well or poorly mattered less than with an air embolism, where mere seconds could be critical.

Obviously embolism classes were desperately needed. So, why didn't they happen? Later, I'll explain why I think they were neglected at the administrative level. For now, we'll look bluntly at why I failed to go to the nursing administration office and recommend such classes. After all, I knew about the problem and understood the solution. I also knew that most of the hospital's nurses had no formal training. Why was I so dreadfully passive?

My excuses start in the next chapter. Just keep in mind that my response was not unique. What I did also explains why many nurses today fear to raise issues they see in their hospital or clinic. The culture often doesn't encourage negative feedback, particularly when it includes an implicit criticism of the administration from which a nurse could face retaliation. That's why coming up with a corrective matters so much. Making needed changes shouldn't depend on nurses making difficult and sometimes risky choices about what to say. It should be easy and natural.

As you'll soon discover, my difficulties are problems that this new senior nurse mentor can solve. Hospitals need someone who is a nurse but isn't working in either a traditional nursing role under the administration or as part of the administrative structure itself. They need someone who can act on her own initiative and authority. That is why I call her a senior nurse mentor, with the emphasis on senior. Extensive experience is a must. So is a love for nursing and nurses. For those who're like that, this job will be a delight.

6. Loyalty to Nurses

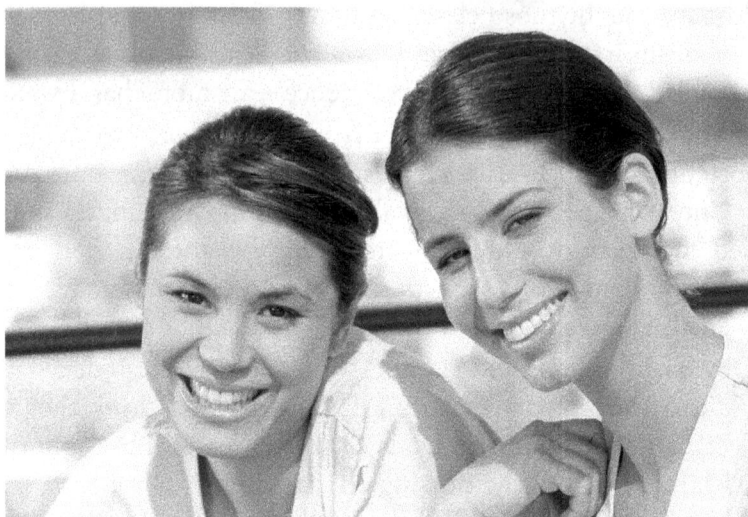

While writing this book, I asked myself why, just after I got off work that day on the teen unit, I didn't go to the nursing administration and ask to talk to whoever was in charge of nurse training. I could have suggested they teach about air embolism and point to my own experience that very day. It wouldn't have been that big a step. I already knew those responsible for CPR training. Whoever I'd talk with probably already knew about me as one of its instructors.

Why I didn't matters because, as we will see, the reasons I did nothing are reasons nurses today often remain silent. **I did nothing because of the loyalty I felt for the nurses that I worked with. People who work together, supporting each other and dealing with common problems, often develop intense loyalties. That's good and should be encouraged.**

That was particularly true in this fourth case of air embolism. The day nurses on the teen unit had it rough—really rough. They were expected to do far too much. When I first began to work there, I wondered why every nurse on the unit was young and pretty. Later, I understood why. Only a nurse who was young and athletic could keep up with the brutal work load. Most were in their mid-twenties and only one was approaching thirty. Those traits almost guaranteed they'd be pretty.

On nights, we had a lot to do, but except for emergencies, circumstances rarely changed. The situation at the start of the shift was identical to that at the end. The fact that nothing had changed in the night was for me an indication I'd done my job well. Because these were serious, long-term illnesses, there were no middle-of-the-night admissions or discharges. Only occasionally did we get a late-night admission with some other illness, and that only happened when we had rooms to spare and thus less to do. That predictability made my work easier. I knew at the start of a shift when a child needed extra attention and could adjust my work accordingly.

Days on the teen unit were never like that. Often, it seemed like the rest of the hospital was conspiring to make our day miserable. There was a steady stream of admissions and discharges. Orders changed. Patients had to be transported for tests and treatment. All might be going well, when suddenly I'd be expected to help with a procedure. Precious time would disappear when I could least afford it. Nurses had it even worse. While a nurse could cover my responsibilities, in the more legalistic world of days, I could not pick up as much of her work as I had done on nights.

Making matters still worse. Tensions between the nursing administration and nursing staff were slowly worsening. You'll find that described in more detail in *My Nights with Leukemia*. On the medical unit, I'd written off the early signs of those tensions, seeing them as confined to our unit and due to an ill-tempered head nurse and two older nurses who resented the younger and more talented second set of new night nurses.

That seemed confirmed during my first months on the teen unit when all went well. Little did I know that the gentle nurse who was filling in for the assigned head nurse was shielding us from unpleasant pressures.

When the permanent head nurse came back, the situation turned sour quickly. She said that all was not well on the unit. I suspected she was playing a bureaucratic game. She had been gone, therefore, she had to claim that matters had been bad in her absence. She was back, therefore the situation had to appear to get better. That's one way to impress administrators.

I disagreed. I could see little that was wrong other than an almost impossible workload. Her hints that some nurses would be fired and her efforts to get me to inform got nowhere. I made a resolution not to say anything negative about a nurse come what may. They were doing their best in a difficult situation. None deserved to be fired.

Her efforts to scare me also got nowhere. I don't intimidate. She claimed that nursing assistant positions like mine were to be eliminated. That made no sense. As assistants, we were busy doing what was expected of us. Would the hospital eliminate our positions and assign our work to more highly paid nurses? I didn't think so.

Worst of all was the impact that criticism had on nurse morale. The administration seemed to feel that nurses weren't motivated. I disagreed. During my time at that hospital, I never ceased to be amazed at just how dedicated all but a few nurses were. They varied in training, skill and experience, but only a few of the many dozens that I worked during those 26 months weren't doing their best.

Looking back, I realize that sufficient on-the-job training was a major issue. There wasn't enough of it, and the situation was getting worse. The lack of air embolism instruction that I've mentioned was a symptom of a much larger problem.

Those tensions had another harmful impact. Motivated nurses want to do good work and don't respond well to criticism. Unfortunately, that criticism meant *more* stress and mistakes rather than *less*. That is why I put that quote from Florence Nightingale on the title page: "How very little can be done under a spirit of fear." She's right. In nursing, fear is a poor motivator and typically does more harm than good.

There was another factor with that fourth embolism I discovered. The nurse I was working with that day wasn't on the teen staff. She was a float, there only for a few days. That increased my sympathy for her. Her mistake—she was the reason for that air embolism—was easily explained by the unaccustomed work load. I knew I could not bring up the problem to administrators without bringing up her mistake. That I did not want to do, so I chose to protect her. Keep in mind that I liked almost all the nurses I worked with. It was natural to want to shield them from such a harsh and critical environment.

I hope you are getting a hint that a senior nurse mentor would work outside that nursing chain of command and thus not be subject to its pressures, particularly the often dysfunctional requirement to record and punish mistakes rather than use them as teaching opportunities. In that environment, the mistake this nurse made wouldn't become a black mark in her official file. It'd be a learning experience. Not repeating a mistake is what matters, particularly when no harm is done, as with that sixteen-year-old girl.

If the hospital had a senior nurse mentor like the one I'm suggesting, I could have talked with her in private, told her what happened, and suggest she ensure that nurse learned about air embolisms. The nurse would learn what she needed to know without getting a bad mark on her record. It's be a win for everyone, especially patients.

Instead, my response was weak and tepid. Yes, I told that nurse what I'd done to respond to that air embolism, but neither she nor I had time to walk through the steps and make sure she got them down right. Remember, I was just a nursing assistant.

A senior nurse mentor would be different. She would have the authority to act. On her own initiative, she could contact that nurse and suggest a meeting, perhaps during lunch or before/after her work. For her part, the nurse would know that the training was off-the-record and for her benefit. We need to be practical. What was past was past. What mattered was that she learn and not that she be punished for a mistake that was only partly her fault.

I've described my failure to act in this chapter. In the next I'll illustrate the limitations I was working under. Pushed to the limit by my assigned responsibilities, I did not have time or energy for much else. There was just so much of me.

7. Just so Much of Me

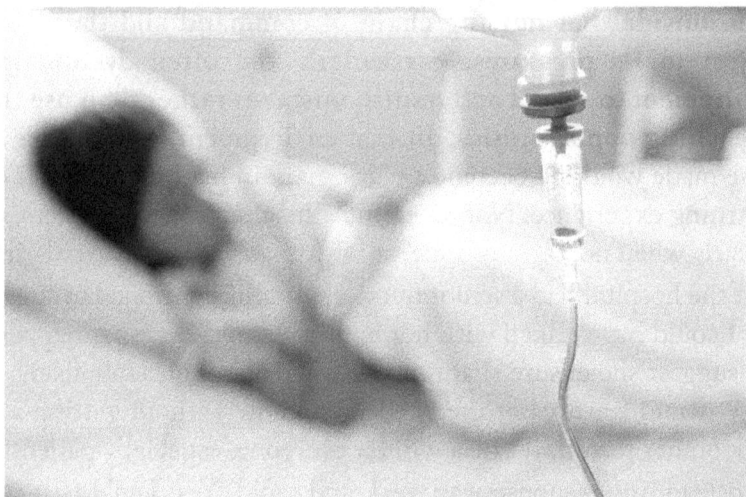

Loyalty to the nurses I worked with was one reason I didn't do anything that could be construed as a criticism of them. There's another reason why I didn't suggest embolism training to the nursing administration. You might call it tunnel vision, but that doesn't quite describe it. I wasn't blind. I saw what needed doing, but still didn't do it. It was a matter of priorities. **To care for my patients, I could not take on a head nurse much less the entire nursing administration. There was only so much me. I could not do more.**

I learned that on the job. When I first began to work on Hem-Onc, I realized that the lives of its children depended on my doing everything right. One mistake and a child might die. There's nothing that can lend clarity to your thinking like that. The result was a personal commitment that overshadowed all else. Other events paled in the light of giving each of those children the best possible chance of life or, failing that, the best possible death. Those kids were my responsibility. Everything else was secondary—everything.

So when two day nurses, aided and abetted by the head nurse, became critical of that second and quite talented new set of night nurses, often harshly attacking them at morning report, I felt sorry for those nurses and tried to encourage them that they were doing good work. But in the end that conflict shaped my behavior only to the extent that it put children at risk. I could fight only so many battles at once. Unfortunately, still intimidated by their first job, those nurses lacked the confidence to fight back.

I was in a similar position. Never forget my limited influence in the hospital's pecking order. I wasn't an administrator, executive, or physician. I wasn't even a nurse. I was a mere assistant. The only people lower than me worked in housekeeping.

Complicating matters, my work was demanding. What energy I had left was not enough to engage in a brutal and exhausting battle with two day nurses that I crudely thought of as being "something that rhymes with witches," much less a head nurse who would support them. Rightly or wrongly, I felt I faced a brutal choice. I could focus on those kids who needed me, or I could join that battle between night and day nurses. I felt I couldn't do both. I chose to keep my attention on the children. Throughout those long and lonely nights I was their lifeline. For that, no one could replace me.

When I moved to the teen unit, there were no nurse-on-nurse battles and never were. That's one reason why I transferred. Instead, I experienced a different frustration that hindered my ability to act. Kind as the nurses I was working with were—none deserved that terrible 'rhymes with witches' label—I faced a problem that I was never able to solve, a most unfortunate one. It involved empathy. Those I was working with did not take newly diagnosed leukemia patients as seriously as I thought they should.

"Why should they?," I reminded myself. A teen newly diagnosed with leukemia doesn't look sick. Typically, the symptom was a mere flu that wasn't going away. Burdened with caring for so many patients, these nurses slighted them. A teen with leukemia was seen as a complication. The tests, procedures, and isolation they required were a heavy burden on an already overworked staff.

Time didn't improve matters. Teens with leukemia were assigned willy nilly to any of the unit's private rooms. Nurses rotated between three clusters, never spending much time caring for a particular boy or girl with leukemia. They never formed the close attachments that Hem-Onc created between patients and staff. Still worse, the later realization that these teens stood a serious chance of dying led some nurses to keep their distance. Busy as they were, they had little time for painful emotional attachments.

I could not help feeling differently. My Hem-Onc experience had burned deeply into me. I felt the plight of these teens much like I had that of their younger counterparts. For sixteen months, I seen children come in appearing healthy. I seen them blasted with chemotherapy because to do otherwise was a death sentence. Then I'd seen some relapse and die in a depressingly short time. The teen unit's slighting of patients with leukemia frustrated me no end, and that complicated my work. I was sometimes angry.

Still worse, teen leukemia patients faced additional complications. First, those teens understood far better than any child would that leukemia meant the possibility of dying. Second, our treatments worked best with small children. I never heard the actual statistics, but I always assumed a teen patient's chances of being alive a year from admission were about 50/50. Someone facing those odds deserves all the kindness possible.

I did all I could, but that wasn't much, and it added to my burdens. Given my own rotation from cluster to cluster, they were never my patients for long. In my head, I flayed about, but I saw nothing I could do. I had to grit my teeth when I saw mistakes—serious mistakes—made because the treat-every-teen policy of the unit meant that few nurses learned the nuances of caring for leukemia.

Yes, failure-to-train was rearing its ugly head again. Having a senior nurse mentor would have been a god-send. I could have talked with her, and she might have found ways to correct the teen unit's deficiencies when it came to leukemia. As a mere assistant, I could do nothing. That wore on me.

I also knew that I was shaped as much by my experience as these nurses were by theirs, that I had similar empathy failings. At various times, I had three patients with anorexia nervosa. Their cases were serious enough that they had to be hospitalized and—with bodies that were little more than skin and bones—those girls looked worse than children with leukemia did after chemotherapy. Long-term, their chances of dying probably weren't that much less.

But I didn't feel for them like I did for those with leukemia. Yes, I got angry. But I got angry at them. Bringing one of them a lunch tray that was typically skim milk and a green salad without dressing, I felt like screaming, "Eat!" Fortunately, there were strict rules never to talk about food with them. Intellectually, I knew that they couldn't see their terrible situation. Emotionally, I thought they were just being stupid. As a result, I wasn't as sympathetic as I ought. The problem others had with leukemia, I had with anorexia. Stresses like those wore me down too.

To their credit, some of the nurses I worked with understood those girls far better than I. One even told me that when she'd been their age she'd been bulimic. That made her more understanding than me, a guy who couldn't understand why those girls obsessed over food.

That's why, for all my fury about the unit's relative neglect of teens with leukemia, I never translated it into efforts to change the culture. There seemed little point in trying. I wasn't in a position to change attitudes or give these nurses a leukemia-specific sensitivity.

The result was dismal. I saw that failure-to-train most clearly when a nurse and a boy's parents got into an argument about his scheduled radiation treatment. For the nurse, radiation treatment always meant a nearby university hospital. The boy's parent knew better. For someone scheduled for a bone marrow transplant, the place to go was that large cancer treatment center, which at that time was one of the few in the world equipped to give whole body radiation. I shuddered when I thought about how upset those parents must have been to discover that their son's own nurse knew so little about his treatment. At its heart, that was a lack of training.

There were other problems that ticked me off—particularly issues with the permanent head nurse. A newly diagnosed teen boy illustrates that. Dan was about eleven and soft-spoken. He and his family had just been told that he had leukemia. They were rushed to us and were admitted early on a Thursday afternoon. I handled his admission. Normally, events moved quickly with leukemia patients, but not so with him. Almost 24 hours after his admission, he had still had not met with any of the specialists who'd be treating him. One resident had dropped by, apologized for the delay, and mentioned that a medical conference was going on at the time. Then he hurried away. That was all.

Seeing how anxious the family was, I grew frustrated. I thought about sitting down with them an offering what advice I could give. After all, there was probably no one on the teen unit who knew better than I what his initial treatment felt like.

I decided not for two reasons. First, there would almost certainly be questions that, not being an expert, I couldn't answer. Besides, Dan's initial tests hadn't been run. At that point in even his physicians knew little. The second reason was more serious. I tried to imagine the uproar that would erupt if I, a mere nursing assistant, had intruded onto the turf of those nationally recognized specialists. Yes, they weren't doing their job because of that rotten conference. But that would make little difference if this issue blew up.

Instead, I came up with what was perhaps a better idea. The teen unit had a closed-circuit television system that could play patient-selected movies. All a patient had to do was request one. Just after lunch, I got the notebook that listed the movies and explained the system to the boy. I even recommended *The Wizard of Oz*. I knew kids liked it because it deals beautifully with facing your fears.

The next day the head nurse called me in for a talk. She wasn't happy, she said, with the time I'd "wasted" explaining our movie system. I should have been changing bed linens.

I wasn't the slightest bit repentant. The time involved, I thought, couldn't have been more than ten minutes and was the only time anyone at our hospital had given the boy and his family during their 24 hours of fretting and worrying. The restraint I displayed amazed me. I wanted to scream at her that she was not only an idiot, but a cold-hearted and callous one. But I didn't. I gritted my teeth and played stupid.

That incident hints at what nurses had to contend with and what I might face if I started raising issues. Some head nurses were capable and talented. But to put it bluntly, others seemed to have moved into administration because they were poor nurses who didn't like patients or their fellow nurses.

Dealing far more than I liked with the bad ones, I discovered that the easy way out was to play stupid. Stupid they understood. Caring about patients was beyond their comprehension. With them, paperwork such tracking as linen changes reigned supreme. If I'd taken on that larger battle, they and I would have clashed with no chance of changing their minds.

To deal with them, I made a choice. Particular incidents where I could make a difference, even though I got criticized, were more important than plunging into a high-level battle where I'd be so over my head I might accomplish nothing. In the case of Dan, defending myself against a head nurse would have also meant criticizing some of the hospital's most senior physicians. It was they, after all, who were delaying that boy's treatment. That could put me into deep trouble and make it harder for me to help patients in the future.

In short, I faced a dilemma. I could help individual patients with specific problems and make a difference, or I could do battle with a system much bigger than I was and perhaps lose. I couldn't do both—or at least so I thought. More on that latter.

Just after I left, the long-simmering clash between the administration and nurses exploded into the open. When the news reached me, I wondered if I'd done the right thing by remaining silent. There were several occasions, including the one involving Dan, when I was so ill-treated by a head nurse, I could have gone to the nursing administration and complained. I'm not sure that would have done anything more than turn the head nurse against me, but it might have given administrators a warning of what was to come. Too much of what the administration heard came from head nurses and too little from a much-put-upon staff. Trouble was brewing.

I did make a parting gift to my nurses. When I resigned to go back to school, I used the letter to complain about the heavy work load on day shift and to suggest moving as much of the work as possible to evenings, where the load was much lighter. Leaving, I felt freer to do that than earlier, when such a complaint might have been regarded as shirking work.

There's a lesson here. My focus had to be on individual patients. They were my responsibility in greater sense than the policies of the hospital or the simmering clash between administration and nurses. I simply couldn't sacrifice my patients for those larger issues.

A senior nurse mentor, on the other hand, would be in a better position to act. Years later, a better response to Dan's situation came to me. Yes, I couldn't counsel the boy or his parents. Working nights, I never even heard that counseling being given. But there were staff members, particularly experienced nurses who worked in the leukemia clinic who weren't attending the conference and who could explain what the family needed to know. Those absentee specialists wouldn't mind their own staff filling in for them.

That idea did not come because my world was severely limited. On nights, I knew almost no day staff. On days, the reason changed, but the result was the same. I was too busy to learn about the rest of the hospital.

That meant when the problem with Dan arose, I knew no one in the leukemia clinic to call on despite having cared for leukemia patients for almost two years. A senior nurse mentor could have made a difference. I could have told her about the problem, and she could have found someone from the clinic. Her knowledge would be far wider than mine and her contacts more numerous.

At this point, perhaps this passage from the journal of John Wesley, founder of the Methodist church, is fitting. Facing criticism for meddling in what some thought were the affairs of others, he responded by explaining what the scope of his responsibilities were.

> I look upon all the world as my parish; thus far I mean, that, in whatever part of it I am, I judge it meet, right, and my bounden duty to declare unto all that are willing to hear, the glad tidings of salvation. This is the work which I know God has called me to; and sure I am that His blessing attends it. Great encouragement have I, therefore, to be faithful in fulfilling the work He hath given me to do.

A senior nurse mentor would have a similar, although more secular mission. Not confined to a particular floor or unit, the entire hospital would be her parish. And yes, she's likely to meet with similar objections to her 'meddling' into what others considered their affairs. Just keep in mind that meddling can be good, particular in confronting that old bugbear, hospital politics. That's next.

8. Hospital Politics

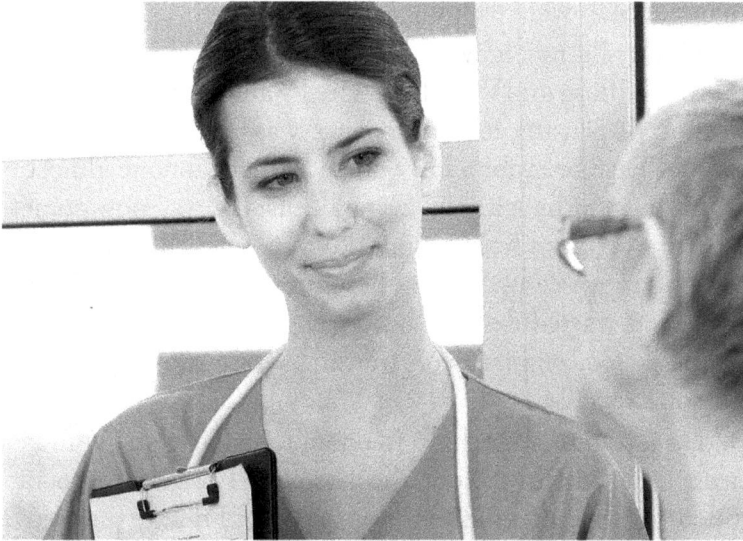

L oyalty to the nurses I worked with was one reason I didn't raise the issue of air embolism training even though I could see the risks. Commitment to specific patients was why I didn't take on broader issues like training and work loads. I couldn't give up my ability to do what good I could for my young patients if I plunged into issues beyond my control. As a mere nursing assistant, I was already punching well above my weight and at risk of being given a bureaucratic put-down.

Politics was another reason I felt boxed in. By politics I mean the various pecking orders and turf-guarding that's ingrained in hospital culture. If I suggested changes, I'd be swimming in the shark-infested seas of those politics. Some might take my suggestions well. Others might say, "Who do you think you are, a nursing assistant, telling us what to do? That's our job." Yes it was, and at times they weren't doing it well.

There was refreshingly little politics on nights. Limited staffing meant everyone had to be practical. The experience that Cala and I acquired meant we carried more weight in decision-making than our lowly rank implied. That was good.

Days were different. For someone who'd grown familiar with the loneliness of night duty, there seemed an overabundance of people on days. That's why rank mattered and professional turfs were heavily guarded. Staff were tripping over one another.

On nights, I'd taken over IVs, so a nurse could go on break. On days, even refilling an IV could be touchy and switching an IV from medication dispensing to maintenance was verboten—as helpful as that would have been for a busy nurse. What I'd done almost every night for 16 months without a single mistake was now something I wasn't to do. That's hospital politics in a nutshell. It often doesn't make sense. I was especially unhappy that most of my Hem-Onc expertise was wasted despite those teens with leukemia. Accompanying the loss of emphasis on training was a growing disdain for on-the-job expertise.

Odd as it sounds, I did have freedom to manage an IV away from the teen unit. Moving about the hospital, I'd come on a mother mystified by why her child's IV was beeping. I'd fix it and move on. All that mattered to that parent was that I knew what to do. Since both parent and I were away from scrutiny, the usual turf rules didn't apply. That's more silliness.

Politics reared its troublesome head in a different fashion one morning, although the issue was isolation rather than an IV. It's good to explain what happened, because it shows that, given the right assistance, I could shape what happened for the better.

Two infectious disease specialists examined a fifteen-year-old girl with shingles, a painful skin infection, and wrote her orders. I wasn't happy that they called for respiratory isolation rather than skin and wound. "She has scabs," I thought. "That's skin."

I knew politics. Technically, I followed the order as given, putting up a respiratory isolation sign and placing a cart with masks and gowns at the entrance. This was day shift and sticklers for the rules were lurking about ready to pounce. Assistants weren't allowed to amend a physician's orders. But I wasn't going to let an order I thought wrong stand unchallenged. Since she was as much my patient as theirs, I practiced *de facto* skin and wound isolation, putting on gloves whenever I went in and washing when I left.

My extra care had a reason, one those experts may not have known. In the room next to her was a teen girl with leukemia whose immune system had been woefully weakened by our chemotherapy. I didn't like the proximity. Placing patients with infections next door to patients with leukemia was one aspect of the teen unit I hated. It was like mixing gasoline with fire.

I went off duty at 3:30 that afternoon, so the isolation order needed changing before then. I had an idea. I knew the infection control nurse, so I called her. She confirmed that indeed the isolation for the girl with shingles should be skin and wound. I then asked her, "Can you issue an order to that effect?" She said she could and would.

I hung up. In a flash, I changed the sign outside the girl's room and added gloves to the cart. One more bit of politics remained. As an assistant, I could take isolation orders, but the nurse would have to write them down. I told her about the change, neglecting to mention what I'd done.

I was taking a chance, betting that those residents wouldn't notice that their order had been amended or, if they did, wouldn't care. After all, the change meant more work for me than for them. By not mentioning what I'd done, I protected the nurse from political fallout. **In the unlikely event that what I'd done became an issue, I'd take the heat not her. I was fine with that. Given the current climate at the hospital, getting criticized was becoming a cost of giving good care. It'd blow over.**

Researching the topic as I wrote this book, I think I understand why those specialists and I differed. Shingles apparently can't infect someone else with shingles. Perhaps that's what drove their decision. But shingles is the recurrence in teens and adults of childhood chicken pox. Being exposed to shingles can give chicken pox to someone who is not immune. By caring for the girl with shingles and then going into the girl with leukemia, I might carry chicken pox. Chicken pox in normal children is typically mild, but in someone with a weakened immune system it could be serious.

Also, chicken pox is extremely infectious. One website claims there is a good chance of getting it if you are merely "in the same room as someone with chicken pox for more than 15 minutes." The real issue was me. I didn't recall having it as a child, so the infection control nurse had me tested. If I'd not had it before, I could catch it and spread it to anyone I contacted who was not immune. I tested positive, so I was safe as long as I followed isolation procedures.

Alas, what I did right with isolation also explains why I didn't do anything about air embolism training. I knew how to get isolation orders changed without getting buried by politics. I knew the infectious disease nurse and that she'd do the right thing. I didn't know how to do the same with air embolism training. The unknown person I talked with might not be the right person. The result might be bad politics rather than good nursing.

By that point, air embolism must have become a touchy subject with the administration. Strange as it sounds, I heard *nothing* about other embolism incidents in the hospital. In fact, far too little was being said about serious incidents of any sort. I had found four patients with air in their lines and one of them had a stroke the next day. That almost certainly meant there were unmentioned incidents with even more serious consequences. The fact that the hospital didn't want to talk about them wasn't good.

True, the hospital was responding. It was spending a large and perhaps unplanned sum to replace otherwise functional IV pumps with pumps that would be better at catching an air embolism. Unfortunately, suggesting another expense, as I would be doing, might not make them happy. Training most of the hospital's nurses might have cost tens of thousands of dollars. I considered that money well spent, but administrators might think otherwise. I had no way to override them.

Here's an analogy that stresses the importance of preparation. Many years ago, while I was studying engineering, I worked at a USAF radar site in Florida that tracked the Mercury and Gemini astronauts, one of three such sites across the U.S. For the critical re-entry phase when they'd be burning through the atmosphere to land in the Atlantic, it was absolutely vital that our radar stayed on track. Giant diesel generators were started up in advance, so there was no chance of losing electrical power. In addition, our powerful FPS-16 missile-tracking radar went into a mode called 'battle short.' Protective circuitry such as circuit breakers were bypassed. If necessary, that radar would continue to operate until it caught fire. Keeping an accurate track on those re-entering astronauts was far more important than equipment worth tens of thousands of dollars.

In a hospital, situations of equal importance occur. The right isolation for that girl with shingles was one example. Training nurses about air embolism was another. Hospitals need someone who is as independent of politics as that radar was of commercial power. If necessary, that person should be able to serve as a battle short, bypassing troublesome delays and getting results quickly. What *must* be done should *always* be done.

In the short term, that might mean doing what that infection control nurse did, changing a bad medical order. It might also mean a senior nurse mentor getting from surgery a list of patients when their central lines were installed and making sure their nurses knew how to deal with air embolisms until the hospital bureaucracy started regular classes.

I hope you see where a senior nurse mentor—given sufficient independence—could make a difference. She'd be like that infection control nurse but for everything involving nursing, particularly morale and training. She could make changes on her own, bypassing politics and operating as independently as that radar did when astronauts made their critical re-entry. That difference would almost certainly save lives. Given all the lawsuits that hospitals face today, it would also prevent mistakes and save money—more than enough to cover her salary. She'd benefit a hospital's 'bottom line.'

In the next three chapters we take up the patient care complications that I faced when I transferred to the teen unit. In addition to problems between nurses and administrators, they illustrate communication issues between nursing staff that a senior nurse mentor might resolve.

These chapters stress that good care isn't just medicines and surgery. Patient feelings matter, including one that is mentioned far less often in nursing than it should be—embarrassment. I take that topic up in another book, *Hospital Gowns and Other Embarrassments*. While written for hospitalized teen girls, what it says is helpful for anyone, young or old, staff or patient, and male or female. The next chapter is about how embarrassment impacts teen boys.

9. Boys Under Siege

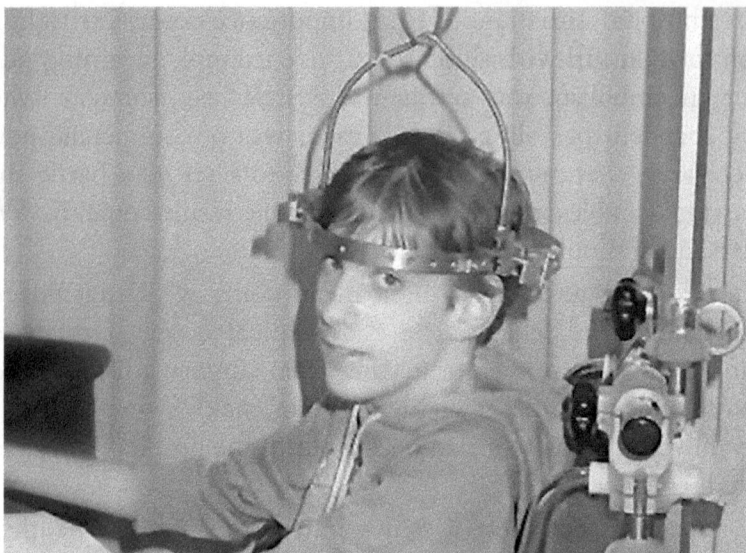

If you've wondered what my teen patients looked like, here's one. He was terrific guy whose back surgery was so risky, the surgeons told him he had a 50/50 chance of ending up paralyzed. Needless to say, I was impressed with his courage and upbeat personality. That's one reason I liked my work. Patients can be great.

As you can tell from the picture, all went well. That was in part thanks to that halo traction, which he could use equally well in bed or out. Screws spaced a few inches apart extend inward from that metal ring into holes drilled into his skull. One of my tasks each day was to do his infection control.

He also illustrates of what I experienced far more rarely than I would have liked on the teen unit, friendship with its teen boys. To explain that requires some background.

Caring for sick children invariably comes with fears attached. My entire time at that children's hospital, I never let go on what might be called the Great Fear. That was the possibility that I'd do or fail to do something that would result in death or injury to one of my patients. That was a constructive fear. I used it to drive myself to work hard and improve my skills.

But there's another fear that comes with starting a new job and might be called the First Fear. It is not necessarily constructive and is often best set aside, since it distracts from what matters.

For Hem-Onc, my First Fear was that my young patients would become terrified of me. I'd seen that happen on day shift during my orientation. With my short white tunic, I'd go into a boy's room and he'd smile. Then a medical technician with her long, white coat would go in, and that same boy would scream. The boy had learned to associate that long, white coat with the pain of a blood draw.

Working nights on Hem-Onc meant that, like that technician, I was closely connected with a child's painful experiences. Would he or she cry or scream when I came into the room? It wasn't a pleasant thought. I had to go into each child's room many times each night. I didn't want to be seen as a monster on the prowl.

Worse still, I *was* connected with pokes and pains. Until we began to use central lines almost exclusively, patient care on Hem-Onc often meant a new IV every two or three days, with me holding while the nurse poked. Even after that became less common, my work still included the horrors of chemotherapy. The timing of our 24-hour infusions often meant that the dose reached toxic levels about one or two in the morning, resulting in vomiting. When that happened, I'd be with the child, holding a small bucket and trying to offer what little comfort I could.

As much as I hated, it, I had a reason to hold that bucket. I did it so a child's parents didn't have to do it, sparing them from being linked in their child's mind with all that suffering. "Better me than them," I thought. Parents agreed. During my entire time on Hem-Onc, I never heard a mother or father say, "No, we'd rather do that."

But would that bad experience mean these kids began to fear and even hate me? That bothered me. After about a month, however, I realized that my First Fear was groundless. They could tell I cared. By some marvelous mental magic, those children didn't connect their suffering with me. Even babies seemed to put the blame where it belonged—on their sickness.

That was wonderfully freeing. Starting with my first night on Hem-Onc, I had resolved to like my young charges and do my best for them. But fear and love don't mix well. Fear of being rejected can keep us from caring as we ought. Now that I knew that I need not fear rejection, I could relax and focus on those kids. They'd smile when I came into their room, and that felt great. I must be doing something right, I thought.

When I began carrying for teens, I faced a different First Fear. I'd transferred to get away from that war between nurses with little thought for what I was plunging into. One of the first things I noticed when I began working with teens was that I had three different patient populations.

The first group was easy to understand. Boys and girls from ten until puberty differed little from the older children I'd already been caring for. They were still kids. With them, little had changed.

The second group, made up of post-puberty boys, was radically different. On Hem-Onc I'd cared for only one teen boy—a fourteen-year-old getting an early bone marrow transplant. My limited experience left me confused. The difficulty was so pronounced that at report when I heard of a new boy who was about twelve, my first thought when I saw him was "Which side of puberty is he?" The distinction wasn't hard to spot and made a big difference in how those boys responded to being hospitalized.

The result was sad. Almost all the post-puberty boys I cared for were morose and withdrawn, so much so that I was never able to build relationships with them. For someone who liked getting to know his patients, it was frustrating. I was never able to break down their walls.

One reason for their unhappiness was obvious. For teens, embarrassment is the equivalent of pain in children. Most of the teens I cared for endured pain stoically, knowing it was necessary. They were less happy about the embarrassing situations hospitals create.

As a result, if these teen boys weren't in a coma or drugged into oblivion, they guarded their privacy with impressive tenacity. Every one wore his undies, with his gown tucked in and his sheets pulled up. Their privacy was under attack, so they reacted accordingly. They fought back as best they could, as little as that was.

I suspected the reason lay with the staffing. Before my arrival, not only did those teen boys have to deal with a nursing staff that was all female, the staff they had made adjustment especially difficult.

I've already mentioned one reason—that every nurse on the unit was young and pretty. These unfortunate guys not only had to deal with their lives being invaded by nurses, those nurses looked like cheerleaders they'd love to date were they not in a hospital. For a seventeen-year-old guy, that was frustrating. You can't impress that cute nurse when you're stuck in bed as helpless as a newborn kitten.

Nursing assistants didn't help. Most were middle-aged women returning to work after raising a family. They were the age of these boys' mothers. What teen boy wants to ask his mother for a urinal? None. In short, being cared for by cheerleaders and mothers was dreadful for these boys. For bed-bound boys, embarrassment was the adolescent equivalent of a child's IV poke. They hated it.

At first, I thought I'd make a difference, but that was only partly true. Although they didn't become less withdrawn when I was assigned to their cluster, they did take advantage of having me around. When I entered their four-bed room, often two or three guys would ask me for their urinals. Not wanting to ask either a cheerleader or a mother, they'd endured the long wait until I came.

Even exceptions proved the rule. You saw one with the picture at the start of this chapter. They were teen boys with major disabilities who'd grown accustomed to intrusions and powerlessness. All the friendly relationships I established with post-puberty boys were with them. They were the one ray of light in the darkness.

That even shaped the pictures I took. In that more relaxed era, I sometimes brought a camera to work. On Hem-Onc, the boys and girls are about 50/50 in my pictures. No so on the teen unit. There I took pictures of boys with major disabilities and girls. Those were the ones I knew well enough that I wanted to remember them. The other boys were a blur.

Alas, during my ten months with teens, I never broke down the barriers those teen boys had raised. I understood the basic problem with their female caregivers and suspected the nurses I was working with might have made matters worse. But I had no answer. The result was the only major care-giving problem I never solved.

How did these nurses make matters worse? Ponder for a moment their plight. Sally the Nurse, cute and lively, is five-foot-two and weighs about 110 pounds. She's got medical orders to do something intrusive with husky Sal the Jock, a six-foot-four, 220 pound high-school quarterback. If he resists, her job become impossible, so she rushes in and pounces, flipping aside his gown and whatever. That's enough to make any guy paranoid.

The nurses had another problem with the boys that I didn't face with the girls. Even with me and thus with no embarrassment issues, teen boys tended to be so uncooperative, I sometimes had to nag them to get compliance with a doctor's orders. In contrast, even with all the embarrassment issues, most teen girls seemed naturally helpful and cooperative. That meant that I had it easy with the girls, while the nurses didn't with the boys. That's why I want to be careful about blaming them. Those boys really were difficult.

Here's the lesson to be drawn from this chapter. Who could I ask about these unhappy, withdrawn teen boys? I couldn't ask the nurses I worked with. Without intending to do so, they were the problem. Asking them would only hurt.

That's where a senior nurse mentor would have been a help. She'd be a nurse, but not one of those I was working with. Her advice about making the plight of those boys easier would be based on years of experience rather than my pitiful few months. She might even persuade those teen nurses to be a bit less aggressive. I knew no way to do that.

So sadly, I failed those teen guys. My frustration with them did have one good result. It heightened my concern for getting along with my remaining patients. Keep in mind that I liked all my patients. They were the one bright spot on day shift. Without them, my work would become a boring, repetitive grind.

The sunny side is next.

10. GIRLS IN SUNNY ITALY

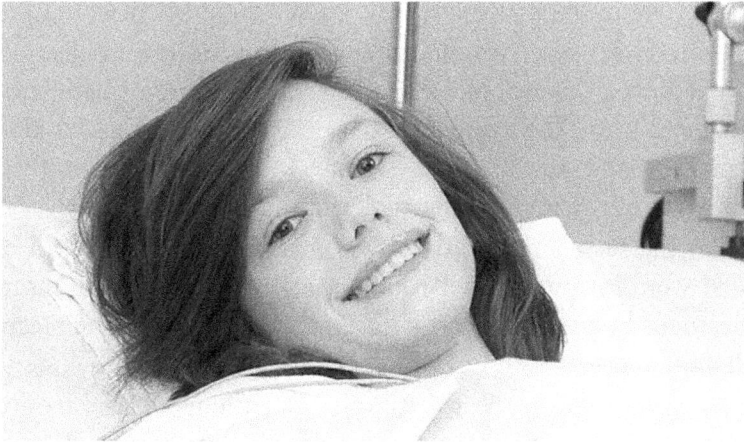

On Hem-Onc, my First Fear had been that pain would cause little children to withdraw and become afraid of me. On the teen unit, my First Fear was linked to embarrassment. I've already given the boy's side. This chapter is about the girls.

I did have one stroke of good fortune. Unlike teen boys, I wasn't new to caring for teen girls. When I'd worked Hem-Onc, we had occasional overflows from the teen unit. All were girls, probably the result of a rule that sent girls to the medical unit and boys to the surgical unit one floor up. Usually, it'd be a girl who'd be with us for but one night. Only Christy, dying of a brain tumor, was an exception. You can read about her in both *My Nights* and *Hospital Gowns*.

Newly employed and working on Hem-Onc, at first I treated these teen girls like children since that was all I knew. But then a situation arose—the Maria I write about in *Hospital Gowns*—when it penetrated my thick skull that I shouldn't treat a fourteen-year-old girl like a four-year-old boy. From then on, I wrestled with what to do. I learned more with each new girl, and was surprised by how different they could be.

As time went on, I began to realize that embarrassment didn't just involve teens. The older kids also had issues. Chemotherapy means fast IVs and constant potty calls. For the younger ones my work was an endless series of diaper changes, bedpans and urinals to spare tired parents a middle-of-the-night wakeup. If I hadn't known how important fluid monitoring was for our critically ill children, I would have hated it as mere busy work. I wanted my work to matter.

From about seven on, my patients began to show modesty. When I went into an older child's room, I'd often find a filled bedpan or urinal waiting. These kids were waking their parents for that. My hunch is that it wasn't sexual—it happened with boys and girls—but was part of growing up. They were acting more like adults.

On the teen unit, calling for a parent wasn't usually an option. Most were in four-patient rooms that had space for no more than brief visits by parents. Fortunately, most could get to the room's tiny toilet for themselves. They didn't need my help.

Now we turn to the third group of patients on the teen unit—those girls. On a typical day, I cared for four boys and four girls, each in multi-bed rooms, along with two or three patients in private rooms. I'd usually stay with that group until my two-day break came and then return to a different cluster.

One part of that work made my head spin. Leaving the boys' room for the girls' was like traveling between two different countries. If you think of the boys as living in a glum northern country where the sun never shines, then the girls lived in sunny Italy.

When it came to dress, the girls were as relaxed as the boys were uptight. Going into their room was like visiting a slumber party. Sheets were kicked down and gowns were never tucked in. Climate control at the hospital wasn't perfect. Hem-Onc, extending out in a long wing by itself, tended to get so cold on winter nights, I often had to get an extra blanket for sleeping children. In summer, the teen unit tended to get too hot during the day. By afternoon, even a sheet could be too much.

Alas, the casualness of the girls created issues. Often, the nurse or I had to catch a girl about to go into the hall and pin up the back of her gown, lest she flash her undies as she walked about. That never happened with boys—never.

In short, most of these girls were as casual about their dress as the boys were uptight. To understand why, simply flip what had the boys upset. Having all female caretakers soothed the girls for much the same reason it alarmed the boys.

Now you can see what my First Fear with them was. Those girls, I told myself, were casual because their caregivers had all been women. Now that wasn't true. I had arrived, manly beard and all. Would my guyish presence change their mood? Would they become as glum and withdrawn as the boys? I hated day's busy work, but felt it was compensated for by more opportunities to know my patients. Unfortunately, I wasn't getting to know many boys. Would embarrassment mean the girls became distant too?

The good news was that I'd learned some lessons on Hem-Onc, lessons not all that different from dealing with pain in little children. I knew I needed to win their trust by being as gentle, careful, and predictable as possible. I must see myself as their guest and act accordingly.

Fortunately, when I started in the spring, I had it easy for a few weeks. Almost all my female patients could get up and about, so embarrassment issues were few. Surgery was an occasional exception. A girl might have had an abdominal surgery with a site on her tummy that needed to be checked for two days post-op. Nurses tended to be aggressive about that. For such checks, they would charge up, flipping a girl's gown well above her waist. They claimed, as one told me, that they needed to "see everything."

I suspected these girls didn't want me seeing that much, so I took a more cautious approach. That mattered because for many of them their first contact with me came before breakfast when I did vital signs and checked their surgery site. Remember, I wasn't concerned with what I could get away with, which was probably a lot given how intimidating hospitals are. I wanted these girls to remain relaxed and confident. I wanted happy patients not morose ones like the boys I was caring for.

As a result, I was careful. Many such patients had a suction chamber draining their surgery site and hanging beneath their bed. I made a rule to check that first. That gave the girl time to adjust to this strange guy poking about her bed. Then I followed that drainage line up to her, pealing back just enough of her gown to check for bleeding or redness at the incision. That, I hoped, would leave the girl feeling safe and in control. That proved right. Their happy little slumber party continued.

Then summer surgeries began. When I started on the teen unit in early May, fellow staff were already talking about the approaching rush in serious orthopedic surgeries. Many required weeks or even months of recovery, so scheduling them in the summer—starting with the most serious—gave these teens time to recover before school started in the fall. At that time, we did so many of these surgeries that "orthopedic" was a part of the hospital's name.

Alas, my first experience with such a patient wasn't pleasant for either she or I. Her surgery was so serious, it came before school was out. I call her Min in the first chapter of *Hospital Gowns*. She was Asian, about twelve, tiny, and terribly shy. Her back surgery was so delicate, she was in a body cast extending from just above her knees up to her neck and out to her elbows.

My job was to come to her every two hours and flip her over, so she didn't develop sores. If she was on her back, I flipped her onto her tummy. If she was on her tummy, I flipped her on her back. It sounds simple but wasn't.

That flip terrified both of us. My fear was medical. Remember that most of Min's body was as stiff as a board thanks to her body cast. She was helpless. Her bed was just wide enough that, if I slid her to the far side, when she came down after flipping, she'd be at the edge of the bed on the near side. As I rotated her, I was terrified that her cast would slip out of my hands, flop back to the far side and tumble off the bed. Clattering onto the floor in such a fragile state might leave her paralyzed for life. That'd be my fault, which was scary. Thinking about bad consequences was how I avoided mistakes. I imagined dangers and prepared.

Min was afraid for a different reason. For a couple our hours each day, she was taken out of that cast by a post-op nurse, so it could dry out. As you might expect it had openings in the usual places. That's what frightened her. When I came up to her bed for those flips, her lovely dark Asian eyes filled with terror.

Some of her terror came because I was a guy. I say some, because I knew what the women caring for her on other shifts did. That sheet, which was her only covering, would be swept aside and only restored afterward. That was practical. Half my fears of her slipping came because I had to adjust that sheet carefully as I turned her. Pulling that sheet off would have made the flipping easier.

For that shy little girl, having a woman doing the flipping made only a small difference. Nothing but a yellow curtain separated her from unexpected visitors. Someone on staff might burst in at any moment. Making matters still worse, her bed was next to a large picture window over the hospital's main entrance. She had good reason to be frightened.

Unfortunately, for all my care I didn't ease her fears. Every time I came to her—three times a day for several days—she was terrified. Looking back, I realize I should have talked to her, promising to handle everything just right.

Why didn't I do that? The reason would torment my entire time on the unit—because embarrassing situations are also emotionally intense situations. If I said something, I might say something wrong. My first attempts at communication were likely to be clumsy, so I didn't make them.

Only later did I realize that there was an answer. Some of my patients were marvelously socially skilled. Whatever I'd said, they would take it graciously. They would have given me the practice I needed. Then I'd have the confidence to speak in touchy situations where it really mattered, as with Min.

Again, that's where a senior nurse mentor would have helped. Asking the nurses I was working with what to say would have been an admission of weakness. I was too proud to do that. They were people I had to work with every day. But a senior nurse mentor who was only occasionally around would be different. I could afford to appear confused and clumsy in front of her. I know that because I never had a problem asking questions—even stupid ones—of the nurse specialists who passed through the unit on their rounds.

Now we look more closely at that summer surgical rush and its complications.

11. HOSPITAL GOWNS

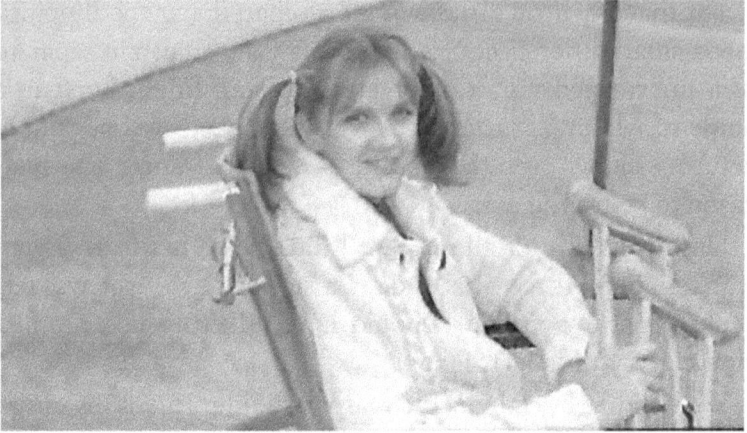

In June, the complex orthopedic surgeries began. Perhaps because I was the only guy on the nursing staff, I spent much of that summer alternating between clusters with boys or girls who'd had those surgeries. I had more strength to move them in bed or to steady them while walking to the toilet.

The boys were in a four-bed room on C cluster. Their problems were often self-inflicted and due to sports injuries or motorcycle accidents. That sometimes meant traction, which left them even more dependent on nurses and hence unhappy. Those who could walk, ever so slowly, to the restroom worried me most. Some were football players so large that, if they'd started slipping, I wasn't sure I could keep them from crashing onto our hard linoleum. I decided I had to be quick to stop a fall before it progressed too far.

The girls were in a four-bed room on B cluster. Their surgeries were often to correct excessive twists in their spine. Even the thought of what that involved—placing two steel rods alongside their backbone and changing how muscles and tendons connected—gave me an enormous respect for them. They were brave.

Their surgeries could last for as long as eight hours. Afterward they typically lay on their back for weeks, occasionally moving from side to side, but unable to sit up. That left them dependent on nursing care, which often meant me. If one of those girls had asked what my work responsibilities were, I could have answered, "Everything you find embarrassing." All too true.

The crisis came with my first assignment to those post-op girls on B cluster. Within minutes, I realized that they and I were in a complicated situation. None had a scrap of clothing under their flimsy gowns. That mattered because most of the techniques I'd developed on Hem-Onc to make care less embarrassing depended on undies.

At first, I blamed the nurses I worked with: "Can't they dress these girls better when I'm around?" Only later did I realize it wasn't their fault. The girls themselves were making that decision. Boys and girls are different. Boys wore their undies with an almost religious intensity because it didn't cause any problems for them when they used urinals. For girls, undies make bedpans a major hassle.

That's why in *Hospital Gowns* I tell my teen readers one of the unfortunate facts of being a patient. In an hospital, I write, you must deal with three great ills—pain, hassle, and embarrassment. Often you can eliminate only two of them. You have to endure the third. Many of these girls considered the hassle of bedpans with undies worse than the embarrassment without them.

Initially, I didn't understand that. My first days of caring for them were like my first days on Hem-Onc, but with embarrassment rather than pain as the central issue. That dread First Fear had returned.

To cope, I adopted a role-playing attitude much like I did when caring for dying children on Hem-Onc. Adopting a role made me less likely to make a mistake. With dying children, my chief fear was that I'd withdraw, make my visits to their room as brief as possible, and not look them in the eyes or get close to them. Those are normal responses, but they're the last things I wanted to do with a dying child who felt fearful and alone in the middle of the night.

So when I went into those children's room, I consciously took on a special role and acted in a specific way. I made sure my visit wasn't hurried no matter how busy I was. If I needed to talk with them, I would crouch down beside their bed and look them in the eyes. I wanted them to know I'd be there for them to the very end.

I took a similarly careful role when I came into these girls' room. I'm a visitor, I told myself, so I need to behave as such. I need to let them know that they are in control. I did my best to win their trust.

I didn't linger, although that mattered little. As needy as they were, they were almost two-thirds my daily work load. I created virtual privacy to make my visits less intrusive. As I worked with each girl, whenever possible I faced away from the others. That made it almost like I wasn't in their room. Last of all, I always glanced away from something embarrassing and didn't stare.

Perhaps the only way I could have been less intrusive would have been to walk around looking down at my shoes and running into beds, chairs, and IV poles. That, I suspect, they would have found amusing and certainly unnecessary. As I soon discovered, these girls were willing to compromise. If I did what I could, they'd accept what embarrassment remained. They clearly wanted to continue living in relaxed, sunny Italy.

After I few weeks, I quit worrying that I'd make these girls as unhappy as the boys. The First Fear passed and I relaxed. Like the Hem-Onc kids, these girls smiled when I came into their room.

But despite that personal success, I remained frustrated with how nursing typically handles embarrassment—primarily by pretending it doesn't exist. I was angry because the techniques I was taught for bed pans and linen changes was ill-suited for some situations. Efficiency and speed were everything. Avoiding embarrassment mattered not at all. That I hated like I hated inflicting pain.

Over the summer, most embarrassment problems resolved themselves. My more clever patients—in *Hospital Gowns* I call them the "sensible girls"—showed me techniques that worked as well as official ones, took mere seconds longer, and were less embarrassing.

That was a relief. Now, instead of being angry that I'd only been taught those speed-above-all-else techniques, I became angry that I'd not been taught alternatives. If you're interested, you'll find them in *Hospital Gowns*. They should be a part of every nurse's training and used with opposite-sex patients. They really do work.

There was, however, one fear involving these girls that never left me. What I had first noticed on Hem-Onc remained true on the teen unit. These girls varied enormously in their attitudes about modesty. Fortunately, I never had another patient as frightened as Min. In fact, I never had another patient who seemed frightened by me at all. I had learned to communicate that they were in control. That freed them to relax and make their own choices.

No, my remaining fear hinged on how some girls chose to game the system. When they needed something embarrassing, they'd wait until just the nurse was in their room and ask her. That's where they were smart. If they'd asked while both the nurse and I were there, most nurses would have said, "Mike will take care of that" and dart away. Then that girl and I would be stuck with one another. Since those clever girls were often among my favorite patients, I didn't want that to happen. I was delighted that, as busy as they were, the nurses were kind enough to oblige them. But I also knew our evasion of the unit's strict division of labor lay under a threat. During that period, the nursing administration was growing increasingly demanding and critical. Our head nurse was one of the worst. In a chapter of *Hospital Gowns* called "Overwhelmed Pala," I illustrate how bad the problem was. It happened just a few weeks after I'd clashed with the head nurse for "wasting time" with Dan.

Pala was in a similar situation to Dan. She was a slender, four-teen-year-old girl newly diagnosed with leukemia. On her second day, I assisted in a spinal tap by a resident so incompetent he failed to get fluid despite three attempts. He stalked off without a word, leaving me to deal with a girl so traumatized, she'd wet herself during the procedure. Her clothes needed changing, and that put me in a bind. My shift was about to end. I'd been behind before being asked to help with the procedure. I was now hopelessly behind. That might make my evening replacement angry enough to talk to the head nurse—not what I needed.

I'd dealt with enough little kids on Hem-Onc who'd wet themselves to know that I had two choices. I could either change her quickly myself, or I could turn around and wait patiently while she did it herself much more slowly.

I knew the former was what I was expected to do. *Speed in everything* was one rule in the hospital. *Staff are not male or female* was another. The head nurse would have no sympathy for this unfortunate girl with a fatal illness any more than she'd had for Dan earlier.

But I knew that turning around and waiting patiently would be a kindness to a girl who'd been through enough suffering in the past two days. I'd spare her yet another humiliation. I opted to risk getting yelled at. What were they going to do, fire me? By that point I was one of the most experienced assistants in the hospital. That seemed unlikely. No, this head nurse would just continue to hassle me. I could live with that.

But there was another risk. Behind my willingness to avoid embarrassing Pala lay a danger that was never far from my mind. If our head-nurse-from-nasty-land found out about that or a similar situation, she might get hot and bothered. Her bad temper was perhaps her only talent. She might issue orders that all the embarrassing assistant work *must* be done only by assistants—meaning me. Of course, both the nurse and I would cheat. But those orders would complicate our little acts of kindnesses.

In fact, the nurses and I were already cheating on an order that came directly from physicians. When I first cared for a girl with anorexia nervosa, a nurse told me: "The doctors have two rules about these girls. First, never talk to them about food. Second, they can't go to the toilet. They must use a bedpan."

The nurses and I obeyed the first order scrupulously. We ignored the second without exception. Given their self-starvation, the bedpan rule might make sense with some patients, but none of ours were that wobbly on their feet. In fact, one got so fed up with her treatment, she dressed in street clothes, walked out of the hospital, and found her own way home. For us, the bedpan rule seemed punitive, so we gave these girls a bed near the toilet and let them take care of themselves. I wasn't the hospital's only secret rebel.

Finally, to be fair, I should mention that behind all their bustle and assertion, the nurses I worked with felt much the same about their care of almost-grown teen boys as I did about the girls. They didn't like embarrassing situations either. On one occasion, a nurse asked me to assist her with placing a urine catheter in a paraplegic boy of about sixteen. I went along, wondering what there was for me to do. There's wasn't anything. She'd just asked me along to make herself feel better.

Another occasion was even more revealing. We had a tall and muscular young black man of about twenty who'd been admitted with a sickle-cell crisis so painful, his pain medication rendered him unconscious. Probably because he felt hot on admission, he had not a scrap of clothing on—not even a gown. Thrashing about in his pain, he would kick off his sheets. As a guy, that mattered not. When I checked in on him, I'd simply put his sheets back in place and move on.

Ah, but in a remarkable display of stupidity, I got ticked off at his nurse. "He's getting a huge dose of morphine," I thought. "She should check on him more often." Yeah, like she really wanted to do that. If I had any sense, I would have put an adult diaper and a gown on him for her sake. Unfortunately, that thought never came to me. At times I could be really thick-headed.

That's where a senior nurse mentor could have served a useful role, serving as a mediator for emotional topics, including making female and male staff aware of the embarrassing complications the other was experiencing with those teen patients. She could have even held a candid discussion on the topic with nursing staff, something the hospital's staid administration would have never considered in a million years.

Next, we look at the role that avoiding controversy of any sort played in my silence.

12. THE COSTS OF CONTROVERSY

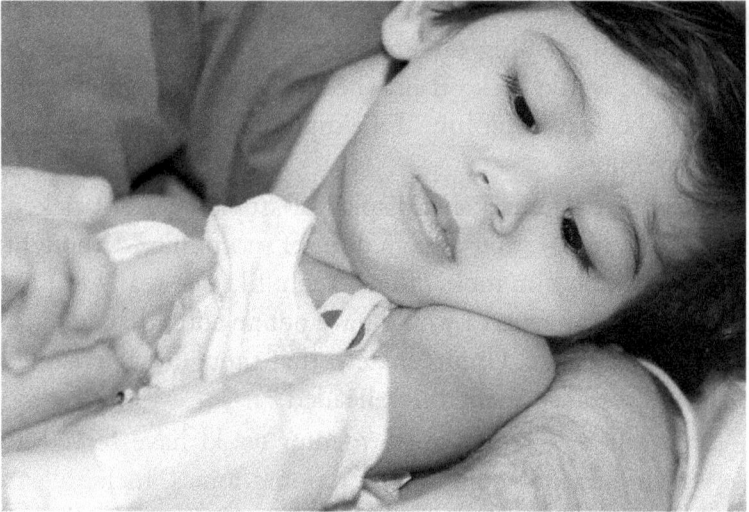

L oyalty to the nurses I worked with, a need to place patients first, messy hospital politics, and the complications of caring for teens despite a hostile head nurse were among the reasons why I didn't act on the larger issues such as the lack of air embolism training or the growing tension between the administration and nurses. It was all I could do, I told myself, to do my job well. I wasn't running the hospital. I was so far down the chain of command, I didn't even have a clear idea how the hospital was run.

There's another reason I avoided plunging into those larger problems. Controversy creates trouble. Creating it might weaken my credibility, something I valued highly. I depended on that credibility to shape decision-making despite my lowly position. Particularly on Hem-Onc nights I needed it to ensure that any concerns I felt about a child would be taken seriously. At the center of my job was watching over those kids through the night.

I deal with that in more detail in *My Nights*, but I'll touch on it here. It's a problem many nurses face. Medicine attaches great importance to numbers. Working nights on a medical unit, my nurse and I spent much of our time collecting numbers for flow sheets kept in bright yellow notebooks. That included fluid in and out, as well as vital signs such as temperature and blood pressure.

After I'd worked on Hem-Onc for several months, I realized there was an aspect to patient care that can't be captured by numbers. A child's mind is sensitive. A change in mental status or personality could signal a problem well before the numbers turned sour. Since I was providing hands-on care while parents slept, I had the best opportunity to spot those changes.

For those intuitions-without-numbers, I needed credibility—lots of it. If I sensed that a patient was in trouble and his or her chemotherapy needed to be stopped or tests run, I had to be taken seriously. Unable to change medical orders on my own authority, I had to persuade others. In *My Nights* you can read about the situations that arose, and how I handled them.

Credibility meant being as error-free as possible. I could not afford to make mistakes, even small ones. During my 26 months at the hospital, I made tens of thousands of decisions. Not all of were right, but none were bad enough to generate an incident report. Why? Because I learned from everything. If I heard about a mistake, I came up with a way to prevent it. If I almost made a mistake, I learned what not to do. If I made a mistake without bad consequences, I made that a lesson. The result was that I never made a mistake that mattered.

That gave me credibility. In the wee hours of the night, based on nothing but a hunch, I feared that I might need to raise such a fuss that phone calls would go out and the issue I had raised would be brought to specialists with years of experience. I didn't want their decision to be distorted by, "Oh, that troublemaker again." Unfortunately, given how people generalize, creating political trouble might damage my credibility on medical matters. Since a child's life might hang in the balance, I felt that I could not afford that risk.

And no, this wasn't about courage. I can be strong-willed when necessary. The issue was knowing when it was appropriate to take a stand. I was willing to risk being fired to get a child's treatment changed. In my mind I saw a giant scale. One side was labeled "A child dies because of delay," while the other read "I get fired for raising a false alarm." Seen that clearly, any risk I make take and any cost I might pay was worth it. I couldn't give a child back his or her life, but I could always get another job. **My real worry wasn't being fired for speaking up. What I feared being ignored when it really mattered.**

Yes, that was an easier choice for me than it was for the nurse I might be working with. I didn't have four years invested in my education nor was I planning a career in nursing. Getting fired only meant the loss of perhaps a week or two of income before I found another job. That was an easy choice to make, especially for kids I liked. The downside was that I would be leaving them behind, but I would never betray them, that was certain.

The difficulty came when I needed to put my credibility on the line in a situation where the indications were vague. One example was Wendy, a patient I will discuss in more detail later. An alarm went off in my mind when I realized that she was doing more than just sleep. She was oblivious to her surroundings. Raising an alarm when she was in trouble was my responsibility. But when I did that, I needed all the credibility I could get.

In contrast, pushing the hospital to train for air embolisms might be a good idea and might prevent something bad from happening, but it wasn't a part of my job like those children were. I carried weight when my patients where involved, weight I could use to influence decisions. I might end up accomplishing nothing if I took on larger issues and was branded a troublemaker.

To have that credibility, I must tread carefully in other areas too. I must get along with other staff, even those ill-tempered day nurses. I had to show good judgments in small matters, so if a situation came up where I needed a nurse to back me up in something serious and fraught with risk, she would.

That was my situation on night shift. My powers were limited. On my own initiative I could have the operator connect me to the sleepy resident who'd been assigned to Hem-Onc that night. I did that all the time. But as a resident, he often knew little. I could go no higher without the agreement of others. That was my difficulty.

On day shift, I faced a different challenge. Since the hospital was fully staffed, expertise was so easily available that even I could simply pick up the phone and call. I didn't hesitate to use that new-found power. I understood all too well how little I knew.

On one occasion, at the end of my shift I was sent to day surgery's post-op area to help a nurse overwhelmed with caring for five small children by herself. One by one, the children awoke and recovered enough to go home with a single exception. A two-year-old boy would not wake up. I knew little about immediate post-op care, and the nurse seemed to know only a little more than I did. At my insistence, a nurse anesthesiologist was called in. On nights, such a person might be a half-hour's drive away. On days, she was just a minute's walk down a hall. She said the boy was fine. I enjoyed having experts on call like that.

Day shift had a problem though. With all the hustle and bustle, patients were sometimes ignored. That's what happened with Lenny, a seventeen-year-old boy, when an accident, probably involving a motorcycle, sent him to our ICU in a coma. When he came out of that coma, he came to us. He was able to look around and respond to what I said but not to speak.

Soon, he improved to the point where he needed better care than we could offer. Since he couldn't complain, I decided on a bold move. Not certain my nurse would agree, I waited until she went to lunch before walking him to a tub filled with warm water. He took to it with obvious delight, rolling from side to side, but taking care to keep his head above the water. It'd been weeks since he'd been able to bathe. He loved it.

I was in luck, first because he didn't drown and second because, while I was with him, his physician came around and was so impressed with his improvement, he promised to transfer the boy to the rehabilitation unit that very afternoon. He was true to his word.

Of course, when my nurse returned, she was surprised to find the boy not in his bed. When she asked where he was, I replied, "Oh, he's taking a bath." From how she looked, you've have thought that I'd decided to drown him to free up a bed. I had to show him happily splashing in the tub, before she'd believe me.

Ah, but to get away with antics like that, I had to be credible, meaning that other staff believed I knew what I was doing. I also had to be creative at coming up with solutions in the midst of all confusion of day shift. That wasn't easy, particularly when I often had no one to turn to for advice.

Think of my plight. When the difficulty with isolation orders arose for the girl who had shingles, I knew the infectious disease nurse and could call her. But when Lenny was being ignored, I didn't know anyone in rehab to contact. I had to come up with that stunt. Lenny and I were fortunate that it worked.

That's where a senior nurse mentor would help. She would be a roving troubleshooter who had what most nurses lack—a knowledge of the hospital structure and personal contacts. The busier the staff are and the more rapidly they turn over, the more a senior nurse mentor is needed. In large hospitals she is a must. Having ready access to good advice like that would do wonders for nursing morale.

Next, we look at how useful a senior nurse mentor would be in a major crisis, including what we can learn from the firefighters who regularly handle such crises.

13. Managing a Crisis

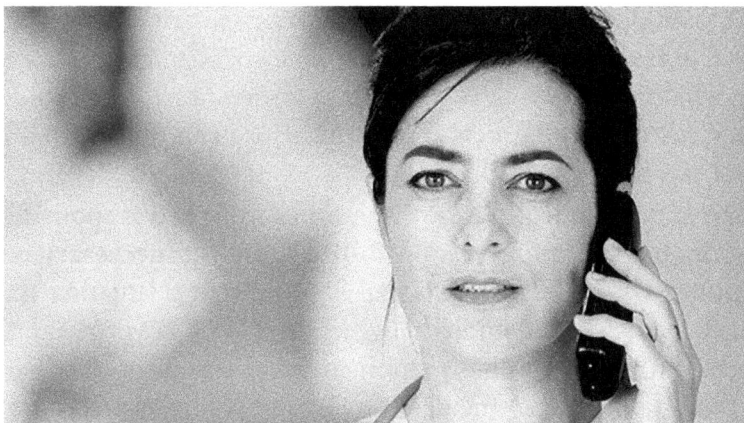

About lunchtime, I was driving across the floating bridge that crosses Lake Washington between suburban Bellevue and Seattle. Halfway across, I noticed a large pillar of black smoke to my northwest. Since the fire creating that smoke had to be over five miles away, I knew it must be huge.

Exiting the bridge near the University of Washington, I headed north for home. It was then that I began to worry. The smoke seemed to be coming from where I lived. Could that be on fire? When I got home, all was fine, but I could see the smoke rising high into the sky to the north and within walking distance. It proved to be a fire in a block-long row of small retail businesses. The area was filled with fire vehicles, firefighters, and hoses.

Have you ever wondered how fire departments manage those large fires? Later, when I worked as a volunteer for an emergency response team based at Seattle's hospitals, I discovered the answer. It's called the Incident Command System (ICS).

Think of a major fire. First to arrive is a fire truck with several husky guys from the nearest fire station. Seeing the situation is bad, they call for assistance and concentrate on making sure everyone gets out of the burning building. As other vehicles and firefighters arrive, the situation grows complicated. In minutes, a fire scene with a few firefighters can grow into one with hundreds. How do fire departments prevent the situation from descending into chaos?

That's where Incident Command comes into play. When someone's workload approaches unmanageable, a division of labor takes place. Responsibilities are formally divided, with each party knowing what their new role is. Because everyone has been trained in the same system, fire fighters from other cities can join them. At that fire I saw trucks from Bellevue.

In short, under ICS, everyone has assigned responsibilities, no one has too many responsibilities, and no necessary responsibility gets neglected. The goal is to prevent a situation that was joked about when I studied engineering: "When you're up to your neck in alligators, it's hard to remember that your original goal was to drain the swamp." Incident Command would assign someone to alligator control, so the others could focus on draining.

Incident Command grew out of necessity and experience. While I was involved in an emergency drill involving the Seattle's hospitals, I talked with a physician who'd come from Japan to study how we respond to disasters such as earthquakes. In Japan, he told me, they usually react by forming a group and discussing the situation until a consensus was reached. Unfortunately, he said, that takes too long. For an emergency, there must be *one person* responsible for specific decisions. A good decision made quickly can be better than a perfect decision made too late.

For instance, if fire fighters are running out of filled air tanks for their respirators, there is someone responsible for that. He can say, "I have a truck with air compressors and tanks coming. It's ten minutes out and will park at the south end of this street." That's Incident Command. Every task has a taskmaster.

Today's hospitals, particularly their emergency rooms, often study Incident Command to prepare for major disasters. Many have brightly colored vests designating who does what, and there are call lists to bring in additional staff when required. That's good.

But hospitals may fail to see a crisis that develops slowly, particularly when they involve intangibles such as training and morale. The result can be like the tale from India about several blind men examining an elephant and coming away with radically different descriptions. One person sees one aspect and acts on that. A second sees another aspect, and acts differently. A third sees nothing and does nothing. No one sees and understands the whole.

That's apparently what happened with air embolisms. We'll look at the parties involved, what each saw, and how each responded.

First were our *nurses*, who were in the front lines of this new technology. Our central lines were so new, most nurses were passing in a few months from having no experience with them to having handled several with no specific training. They were muddling along as best they could. Because those lines worked like peripheral IVs, many thought that was all they were. Typically, they only realized the seriousness of an air embolism when one struck them. That was true in all four of the cases where I was involved. Experience often comes too late as a teacher.

Just above them in the hospital's hierarchy were the *head nurses*. There my experience was limited to two full-time and one temporary substitute, so I can only describe how the two full-time ones responded.

Unfortunately, their response did not impress. They did not seem to investigate the circumstances behind an incident. Instead, they searched for someone to blame, so no responsibility fell on them. Since the primary cause for an air embolism was *their* failure to ensure that nurses received the proper training, I suspect that never entered into their reports. As a result, the real cause of those mistakes was never pointed out from their level. Nurses took all the blame.

Moving higher still, there were the *training staff*. Nurse training did exist. Classes in CPR and other topics were taught, along with an occasional nursing grand rounds. On my own time, I attended training that impacted what I did, whether intended for doctors or for nurses. Attending for free was one of the fringe benefits of my job. Unfortunately, as far as I know, there was never any formal instruction on the new risks created by central lines—none.

Finally, the *administrators* did do something constructive. They looked at the incident reports filtering up and concluded, quite rightly, that new IV pumps were needed, ones whose air sensors could not be misplaced. They allocated the money to replace our existing pumps after a year-long testing period. But they failed to do the one thing that would make an immediate difference—comprehensive training for nurses.

I'm not sure why that was true. Maybe the issue was communication. Perhaps those who were responding to incidents weren't in touch with those who handled training. Perhaps those responsible for training thought a central line was just another type of IV. Despite being one of their part-time instructors, I don't know.

And yes, I could see the whole. Having discovered four embolisms, I knew the problem all too well. In this book, I've offered excuses why, despite seeing the big picture, I did nothing. I certainly should have done better. But keep in mind the extenuating factors.

First, as nursing staff we almost never heard about problems on other units. A air-tight lid seemed to have been placed over all such communication. Even gossip was discouraged. Keep in mind how difficult that made it for nursing staff who, like me, thought through how to avoid every mistake we heard about. What we did not hear about, we could not learn from.

That was true of an incident I describe in *My Nights*. A young woman had heart surgery followed by a terrible blunder in the ICU. Sodium bicarbonate from her IV leaked into her arm, leaving the tissue badly damaged and her arm a sickly slate gray. A few days later, she became my patient, and I tried to discover what had happened. I drew a complete blank. After her surgery, her medical record suggested all was well up to a certain point. After that, it was clear all was not well, but nothing explained what had gone wrong. That's the air-tight lid, and I blame it on lawyers.

A similar lid was placed over air embolisms. As much as I might suspect other embolisms were happening, I had no way of knowing. If the hospital had been more open about those other incidents, perhaps I might have spoken out about the need for training. Their silence led to my silence.

Second, during my 26 months at the hospital, I cannot recall anyone in the administration ever asking me or anyone I was working with for suggestions. Right or wrong, that leaves the impression that new ideas aren't unwanted. The letter of resignation

I submitted about overworked day nurses was the only such action I knew about.

Third, on some but not all units, the head nurses formed an intimidating wall between nurses and the nursing administration. They did not want criticism to flow upward, criticism that might implicitly condemn them. Their hostility prevented nursing staff from discovering if the nursing administration was receptive to suggestions. Maybe it was. Maybe it wasn't.

Even exceptions fit the pattern. The hospital was trapped in a Catch-22. On a unit where the head nurse led well—and I knew of at least one—the nurses had no serious issues to raise and thus no need to communicate past their head nurse, who was herself keeping the administration well informed.

In contrast, on units where there were problems, head nurses did their best to silence any effort to raise issues directly with the nursing administration. Complaints from nurses would reflect badly on them. Even more disturbing, head nurses could take revenge on those who made trouble. That's why my criticisms were included in a resignation letter. Leaving, she could no longer do anything to me.

Behind those communication failures lies a shift in the hospital culture that was so all encompassing, I can only offer a general description here. Parts of a healthy working environment lingered on for a time. One example were those first experienced nurses who went out of their way to teach me good nursing skills. I benefited enormously from that.

But that good working environment was fading. I first noticed the change shortly after the second set of replacements arrived. One night, the nurse I was working with felt that Hem-Onc had more seriously ill children than she could safely handle. She told the other nurses, and they rallied to her side, each taking one or two of the less serious children, so she could focus on the more critical. With the disaster of that first set of replacement nurses still fresh in my mind, I was delighted.

Unfortunately when the head nurse arrived at 6 a.m., she saw the situation differently. When they told her what they'd done, she attacked rather than praised. I was so ticked off, I made a point of complimenting each of those nurses. Later, as matters went from bad to worse, I concluded that what happened that night was my first warning of the trouble to come.

A dangerous shift was taking place between a weak but still cooperative team environment where staff helped each other to a critical, blame-shifting environment in which each nurse was left isolated and afraid. Criticism wasn't simply being added as yet another way to motivate nurses. Criticism was replacing cooperation.

Why? Because nurses who could unite to give better care could also unite to resist unfair criticism. From the point of view of those who wanted to impose blame, that must not be. That growing isolation then became the source of many troubles. It was why nurses would later feel that they had no alternative but to quit.

From what I saw, the only nurses who gained from this shift were the ones who attacked others to divert attention from their failures. The growing climate of recrimination made it easier for them to evade responsibility. In contrast, most nurses were too decent to launch unfair attacks and many were too new to nursing to defend themselves well. At a hospital that liked to hire nurses just out of school, the latter situation was all too common.

That's where a senior nurse mentor independent of a failing system would help. Nursing morale would be her primary responsibility. When morale began to falter, she could act on her own authority. She could study the situation, taking on that destructive climate of fear and criticism and encouraging a return to cooperation and support.

For instance, a senior nurse mentor could listen as nurses complained about a bad work environment and evaluate what they said. She might agreed or disagree, but no nurse would ever be punished for talking with her. Responsible only to the hospital's CEO, she could take whatever action was necessary to turn a bad situation around.

Next we look at the morale-destroying games that haunt many bureaucracies, including hospitals.

14. BUREAUCRATIC GAMES

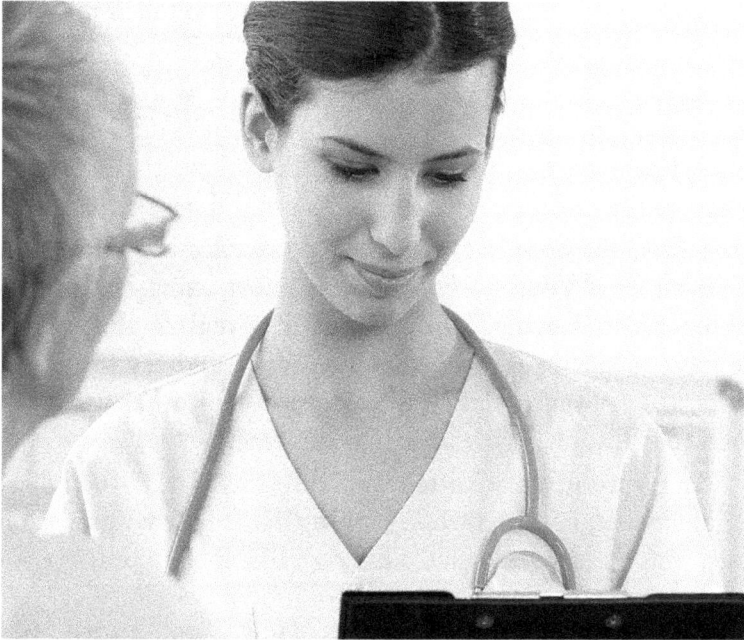

In March, I resigned from the hospital to begin graduate studies in medical ethics at the University of Washington. Many of my courses would be with nursing students and graduate nurses.

Over the summer, I drove up to Canada to attend a medical ethics conference at the University of British Columbia. There I met a nursing school professor and asked her a question that troubled me, "Why do hospitals hire stupid people as head nurses?"

She obviously knew what I meant and didn't hesitate to answer: "Because they want someone who'll do what they tell them to do." Alas, that made all too much sense.

Her reply answered a question that the hospital's chaplain had put to me a couple of months earlier when he sat down next to me at a town meeting being held at one of Seattle's television stations. "Why, he asked, "was there so much tension between the hospital administration and its nurses." The situation had grown so bad, he went on to explain, that 20 percent of the nurses had quit. In addition, he went on, the hospital's reputation among local nurses was so bad, hiring replacements was almost impossible. To keep the staffing up, the hospital had to demand overtime well in excess of their contracts. That did nothing to endear it to the heroic and overworked nurses who remained.

I already knew about the hiring trouble, which happened just after I left. In my classes that spring, whenever I'd mention to a nurse classmate the hospital where I'd worked, their response was along the lines of, "Oh, that terrible place. I'd never work there."

At first, the speed at which those troubles burst into the open surprised me. When I'd left, I didn't know a single nurse who was talking about leaving. **Only later did a realize that when people have minor problems, they complain and try to get change. When they're really ticked off, they look for other work and quit when they find it.** That's what had happened.

Serious problems are often rooted in the past. Although I didn't realize it when I started work, looking back, I get a glimpse of those roots. You've heard one clue, although like me at the time, you may have missed it.

That clue lies with my orientation. Hem-Onc had some of the hospital's most critically ill patients. It routinely cared for children in conditions as grave as those in the ICU. Our children weren't transferred to the ICU because they had become sicker. They were transferred when their care demanded more than two staff responsible for seven children could manage.

For instance, someone with a platelet count of just 6,000—roughly 2 percent of normal—is scarily sick. Caring for such a patient is like entering a warehouse filled with explosives bearing a flaming torch. But if nothing can be done, staffing isn't an issue. We could grimly wait out that crisis as easily as the ICU.

Now recall my situation. I was hired to be half of a nursing team caring for those children at night when expertise is thin. Imagine for a moment that you're my head nurse. You know that my three months of EMT training has little to do with the specialized care on Hem-Onc. You also know that my first week of classroom orientation only covered basics like taking temperatures. Finally, you worry when you realize that you have only three weeks to ready me to take on Hem-Onc at night.

Would you waste those precious three weeks having me work with the medical unit's regular day patients? Would you have me doing work so dull and repetitive that I learned almost nothing after the first few days? I certainly hope not.

Orientation to a job is an orientation to *that* job. I *needed* to be working day shift on Hem-Onc to be ready for nights. I *needed* to spend a few days in the Hem-Onc clinic where kids with leukemia were initially screened, and where they were followed up while in remission. That's obvious, and yet not only did that not happen, I wasn't even told where I would be working. That denied me even an opportunity to prepare myself.

Does that make sense? Not as good nursing administration. But as bureaucratic game playing it makes perfect sense. Here's why.

Recall when the teen's head nurse attacked me for explaining our in-house movie system to the boy newly diagnosed with leukemia? What I did, she said, kept me from changing bed linen.

Linen changes! The day before that boy and his parents been told that he had a cancer that left untreated was 100 percent fatal within mere months. Yet for a full day after his admission nothing happened. Both the boy and his parents were understandably confused. Pitiful as what I did was, by offering that movie I was providing better nursing care than by doing those linen changes, which evening shift had ample time to do.

Demanding busy work to the exclusion of all else was a bureaucratic game that these less-than-capable head nurses often played. My first head nurse made herself look good on paper by using me that way. Bored but busy, I generated 'work done' numbers changing linen and such. That's what mattered to her. Literally *nothing*, I found, trumped bureaucratic appeasement in the minds of some head nurses, not even one of the saddest experiences I had at the hospital. I tell the story in more detail in *My Nights*, but here's a summary.

Susie was a sad little black girl of about eight. She was dying from a tumor that had so wrapped itself around the arteries close to her heart that surgery was impossible. No mother or father ever stayed with her. No family members visited. She was dying all alone.

Susie was too terrified to fall sleep. Each night, I'd hurry though my other start-of-shift work to rock her to sleep. Since I had to make sure she was sound asleep before I put her in bed, that took about 45 minutes.

The time involved was the hitch. I could do that only once and then only by skipping all my breaks and being as quick as possible with my other patients. When Susie woke again in the middle of the night, I could give her no more time. I had six other critically ill children to care for and could not put their lives at risk. That's why one morning I became so frustrated, I wrote in her nursing notes, "Someone needs to stay with her at night."

How did this head nurse respond? Probably alerted to my remark by one of the ill-tempered day nurses, she called me in and berated me for that remark. Her bureaucrat mind didn't like problems coming out and perhaps even imagined that there was a policy against describing serious patient issues in nursing notes. Do you see why I concluded that some head nurses were exceptionally stupid as well as cold-hearted and callous?

Looking back, I wish I'd have scrawled those words in big, bold letters in Susie's medical chart, a place where only physicians typically made remarks. It might have drawn a response. Alas, I didn't. Even worse, that incident came as nursing morale on the medical unit was collapsing, and I was transferring to the teen unit. I let myself get too distracted by that to do more for little Susie. Fortunately, on her on initiative one nurse, bless her heart, did stay with her, holding her and talking to her as she breathed her last. She didn't die alone.

Authoritarian Nursing Administration

At this point, it helps to recall some details from the history of hospitals. Today, we consider hospitals as the best place to be when you are seriously sick. That was not always so. In fact, during the nineteenth century hospitals were typically so terrible—dirty and staffed with drunken excuses for nurses—that only the poor with no other alternative used them. Those who could afford to do so were cared for in their homes.

What brought change were then-new technologies, particularly the X-ray machine, discovered in 1895, and lab-based diagnostic tests for diseases (syphilis in 1903). A physician could no longer carry everything he needed in a black leather bag. Only a hospital could provide those new technologies. Hospitals were soon on the path to becoming what they are today, complex institutions that usually give excellent care.

But no institution remaking itself starts from scratch. Those doing the reorganizing looked around for successful models in other fields and adopted them. In the case of hospitals, for good and ill, their models were the once well-regarded factories of the early twentieth century, such as those run by Henry Ford. They were efficient, they were profitable and, perhaps most important of all, they took people who had grown up on farms and turned them into factory workers. That seemed to be the solution to the staffing problems of these new hospitals, which had to transform hospital nursing and make it no longer be the domain of those too incompetent to succeed in private-care nursing.

That choice had good and bad consequences. Like those factories, hospital work was driven by fixed work schedules. Like factories, the organization was heavily hierarchical, with bosses and supervisors ruling over workers, particularly nurses, who were treated as of limited ability and little different from the tools they used. Because those workers were held in low regard, they were expected to follow orders and adopt standard procedures rather than show initiative and judgment. Behind all that lay an urge to maximize efficiency. Here's how Wikipedia describes the long term impact of what was then called "scientific management."

> Although scientific management as a distinct theory or school of thought was obsolete by the 1930s, most of its themes are still important parts of industrial engineering and management today. These include analysis; synthesis; logic; rationality; empiricism; work ethic; efficiency and elimination of waste; standardization of best practices; disdain for tradition preserved merely for its own sake or to protect the social status

of particular workers with particular skill sets; the transformation of craft production into mass production; and knowledge transfer between workers and from workers into tools, processes, and documentation.

Read my earlier hospital books, and you'll hear frustrations much like those voiced by workers in Ford factories a century ago. Like them, I was fighting back against being treated as a cog in a machine. Working on Hem-Onc, I rebelled at the assumption that I do no more than collect vital signs and sound an alarm when they were out of line. In *My Nights with Leukemia* I describe how I chose a different path. I would understand my patients and use my judgment to detect when something was going wrong well before the numbers went awry.

One situation illustrates that. I'd been off for a couple of days and returned to discover that Hem-Onc now had a baby girl only three months old. She'd be my youngest leukemia patient.

She'd been admitted two days earlier when both the evening and night nurse had been on duty, so little was said about her during report. When I went into her room for the first time I was in for a shock. Her IV was running at 100 cc an hour. I looked at this tiny, sleeping baby and again at the IV. Then I spun around and found the nurse. "Why is that IV so fast?," I asked.

She explained that fast IV was necessary. A baby's kidneys could not concentrate the waste her body was eliminating due to the just-completed chemotherapy. That was also why, to make oft-repeated diaper changes easier, the baby was sleeping tummy down on an open diaper. Finally, with all that fluid going in, trouble would quickly follow if her kidneys could not keep up. That's why I was to take her blood pressure often.

The more I thought about my youngest patient, the less satisfied I was merely measuring blood pressure. I suspected that this baby's body would do everything possible to maintain a stable blood pressure, that her pressure would only go wrong when everything else fell apart. There had to be a better way.

I checked medical and nursing books. They offered several ways to spot fluid overload. Growing puffiness under the skin, I concluded, wouldn't work. Her baby fat concealed that. A gap between fluid input and fluid output was better, but our tummy-on-diaper scheme leaked.

Only the third approach offered hope. That excess fluid would collect in her lungs, changing her lung sounds to crackles or rales. Unfortunately, I'd not been trained to recognize such sounds, so I came up with a fix. Each time I did a diaper change, I would listen. If that sound changed, I would raise the alarm.

Why wasn't I taught about those sounds, valuable as they are? For much the same reason workers in those long-ago Ford factories were only taught rudimentary skills such as tightening nuts on bolts. I wasn't expected to know more. Not trusted to make judgments, I was relegated to charting numbers even when those numbers did not offer the best warning of danger. That made no sense to me. Lung sounds aren't heart surgery. They're easily learned.

In those car factories, demeaning workers led to a high turnover, in some cases over 100 percent a year. Rather than respect workers and find ways to deal with their dissatisfaction, management offered high wages. Workers responded with unions. The result was a morass that still afflicts auto manufacturing. TheHenryFord.org has this to say about the company's enormous 'ore to assembly' Rouge factory outside Detroit at a time when the complex had an incredible 100,000 employees at a single location.

> By 1928, the complex was complete, yet it was never settled [operationally]. The Rouge continued to operate throughout the Great Depression, yet Ford's obsession with ever-increasing cost reductions through methodical efficiency studies made life difficult for workers.

> On May 26, 1937, when a group of union organizers led by Walter Reuther attempted to distribute union literature at the Rouge, Ford security and a gang of hired thugs beat them severely. It would be known as the Battle of the Overpass and became a pivotal event for the United Auto Workers and other unions.

Today, some hospitals have a similar authoritarian pattern—although fortunately without the hired thugs. They regarded rules and metrics—meaning counts of things—as supreme values. The assumption is often that nurses care little about their patients, that they aren't that bright, and that the best way to motivate them is to threaten punishment. In-depth training—such as lung sounds rather than measuring blood pressure—is seen as of only limited value.

I saw that when the permanent head nurse returned to the teen unit, replacing the gentle temporary head nurse. She spent no time watching our nurses work. If she had, she would have discovered just how overworked they were. Instead, she spent hours pouring over nursing notes, looking for what she regarded as mistakes.

One day she called me into her office over what she thought was a serious blunder. Did my patient suffer. Not in the slightest. Was there anything I had failed to do? Not at all. I'd not only given him excellent care, I'd deliberately and consciously done so. I knew my job and had done it well.

The patient was a boy of about eighteen getting what I call in *My Nights* "a chemotherapy drug-from-hell called cisplatin." I hate it like I hate few others things. Under no circumstances would I neglect to give a patient getting it top-notch care. If a patient does not void frequently, it can do great harm. Drugs.com says that renal toxicity occurs in 25 to 36 percent of patients even after a single dose. Think of multiple quarter-sized blood clots in every urine void for months afterward—that bad.

As far as I know, none of my patients suffered those complications. I made sure they had a fast IV and would have yelled bloody murder if they didn't. I remember that particular teen boy's rate to this day. It was 200 cc's an hour—well over a gallon a day. I also followed orders to the letter. Day or night, they voided every two hours. If they had a problem doing that, I got Lasix ordered. I never took chances with that drug—never.

What, you might ask, was her problem with my care? Well, it seems I hadn't noted that all was well in those nursing notes. "Hey," I felt like saying, "we don't document when all goes well. If the patient isn't febrile, we merely record their temperature. If one voids as expected, we record the volume." Good numbers speak for themselves. Nursing comments are for issues needing attention.

Notice something revealing. One head nurse (Hem-Onc) attacked me for putting something of great importance in those notes—Susie's need for a nighttime companion. Another head nurse (teens) attacked me for not putting something unnecessary in those notes, the fact that a teen's care was going well.

That's what I mean by authoritarian and critical. It's obsessed with paperwork and numbers. It treats capable and caring nurses as failures. Since nurses are regarded as unmotivated and incompetent rather than committed but perhaps in need of more training, an extensive orientation and regular, up-to-date follow-up instruction matter little. What matters are heavy doses of criticism constantly repeated. Threats, these people believe, can substitute for training. As a sign I once saw put it, "The beatings will continue until the morale improves."

Recall the orientation I did not receive and the poor orientation given to the new nurses who came along three months later. Notice the sudden verbal attacks with little or no praise for work well done. That was one reason why I considered these head nurses stupid. They did not understand how to manage people. Under their unfair criticism, nursing morale was collapsing.

During my last few months on the job, some nurses were turning to their union for help. But that did not make much difference. As with those earlier auto workers, it merely transformed a hidden conflict into an open one. The conflict itself was not eliminated.

In the next chapter we'll look at the issues behind the conflict. As you read, think about how a senior nurse mentor, operating independent of the administration and tasked with hearing nurse complaints, could make a major difference.

15. Blaming Nurses

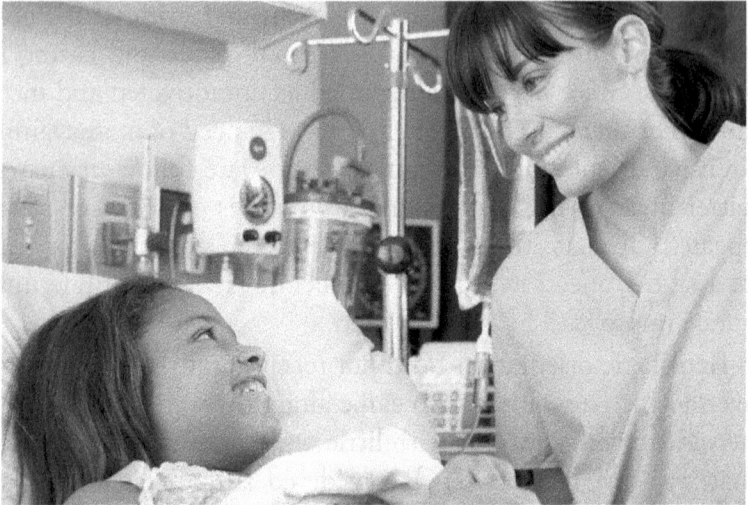

I found it easy to brush aside the attacks from those two head nurses because I knew I was being treated unfairly. Susie did need company at night, something I could not provide. That teen boy did get top-notch care from me. The fact that only criticism either head nurse could level at me was that bogus told me that I was doing excellent work.

But keep in mind that, as an assistant, I had it easy. It was true that when I worked on Hem-Onc I needed the specialized skills those first nurses taught me. One oversight on my part might mean a child would die. I realized that, and the demands I placed on myself were far beyond anything that head nurse even understood.

The teen unit was different. With but a few exceptions such as that cisplatin, most of my work didn't require specialized training—just basic care given with good sense. No one needed to teach me that, when I walked a football player who weighed far more than I did to the toilet, I had to be careful.

On the teen unit the cards were heavily stacked against the nurses. They faced a heavy burden. First was the constantly chang-ing, too-heavy work load they shared with me. Second were the complexities of caring for almost every kind of illness the hospital handled from cancer to surgery and psychiatric. That fell far more heavily on them than me. Third was the fact that some of their mistakes could have rapid and disastrous consequences. They were expected to do all that with little or no support from the administration. That was most unfair.

I saw that one late one morning when the nurse I was working with mentioned she was worried about an order to give vitamin K via IV to a cystic fibrosis patient who normally took it by pill. She recalled from nursing school a risk in vitamin K given that way.

I knew nothing and could be of no help. Medications were where my limited formal training showed up most acutely. When I returned from lunch, I found that disaster had been narrowly adverted. The girl had reacted to that vitamin K. Forewarned, the nurse responded well.

Ah, but that nurse was one of the hospital's most capable. She was a delight to work with and would be on the short list of nurses I would want caring for me were I sick.

Other nurses might not have recalled those dangers from a nursing class years earlier. Was the hospital giving those nurses any help? Not really. Did a warning accompany the dose? No. Was the hospital scheduling classes on drug reactions and overdoses, perhaps taught by a staff pharmacist? Not that I recall. If there had been, I would have attended. I was aware just how little I knew. Was there someone to contact when a nurse had doubts about a medication? No, although a savvy nurse could call the pharmacy.

But woe betide the nurse who made a mistake, even one that flowed—as in the case of that vitamin K—from a physician's ill-considered orders. That particular nurse escaped criticism by being prepared, but not all nurses were as sharp as she.

That was becoming the hospital's core problem—an authoritarian atmosphere dominated by intense criticism and devoid of adequate training or support. That's what the nursing staff was enduring. That's why many finally said, "Enough!" and left.

I mentioned it earlier, but the incident fits here too. Near the end of my time on Hem-Onc, the night nurses were extremely stressed out and fearful of being attacked at morning report by day nurses egged on by the head nurse. People under stress think poorly, so one night a nurse did not notice that a morphine order for a boy was ten times what it should have been. The boy almost died.

Just minutes after that overdose, I heard the night-shift supervisor giving the nurse helpful advice. Learn the usual doses of common drugs, she said, and question any that seem out of line. That was well and good, but formal training should have taught her that *before* this incident and been constantly repeated. What came was too little too late. For me that incident was the final straw. Unable to fix Hem-Onc's now rapidly worsening morale, I decided to transfer.

Realistic and Supportive Nursing Administration

WE TURN NOW TO a view of nursing administration that's realistic and supportive rather than authoritarian and critical. Rather than treat nurses as incompetent and poorly motivated, it takes them as they are and helps them become better. It recognizes nurses are human, differing in their abilities, and that those differences should shape policies in ways that support nurses rather than crush them. One factor is a realization that, loosely put, there are three different types of nurses.

1. Exceptional Nurses

The first group of nurses are the exceptionally capable. Taught ten skills in class, they learn a dozen because they link those skills with others. Taught in nursing school that patients can react badly to vitamin K given by IV, they'll not only remember that, they'll create a well-remembered list of drugs that should be given with care.

If you're sick, you're fortunate to have exceptional nurses. They teach themselves, striving to be better and, as a result, outperform their environment. Even in a bad system, they give good care.

One of the nurses who provided my initial mentoring was exceptional. I was so impressed, I did my best to adopt her attitude. I never grew complacent. I learned constantly. I questioned even the slightest change in my young patients. When I heard about a mistake, I did not rest until I knew how to avoid making it myself. If something needed to be done, I did it. Most important of all, I constantly reminded myself that a mere inconvenience for me might mean life or death for some child.

Remember what I wrote about an authoritarian system that assumes nurses aren't that bright? That attitude is loathed by these talented nurses. Hospitals often fail by not giving them enough scope for their talents. Some get so frustrated that they leave nursing altogether, which is a great loss. Hospitals need nursing positions that are as great as nursing talents. Those positions should not all be administrative. These people are too talented *as nurses* to be wasted on paperwork.

Where I worked, the exceptional nurses often moved into specialty areas such as treating diabetes, where they could make decisions on their own initiative and avoid niggling bureaucrats. That was good for patients with specific problems. But it was not good for the hospital as a whole. It diverted talents that could have been used to improve the skills of other nurses.

Taking advantage of the skills of these exceptional nurses is why hospitals should have senior nurse mentors. They need gifted nurses who operate outside the usually administrative boundaries and can act on their own authority and initiative.

In fact, my relationship with those specialty nurses was much like that I'm advocating for senior nursing mentors. When they passed through the teen unit on their rounds, I asked them questions. No matter how stupid those questions were, they gave helpful answers. I was impressed and learned a lot.

My initial experience also illustrates that mentoring works. Recall that I started Hem-Onc as a virtual zero, knowing nothing about the care I was to give. My EMT training was irrelevant. My month-long orientation was worthless.

But thanks to my apprenticeship with those first nurses, I learned how to handle Hem-Onc, including its complex IVs and dangerous air embolisms. On my own, I went one step further. I combined those last two skills into a third. I used my flashlight to check IVs every time I entered a darkened child's room. That's the proper way to learn. Learn two skills so well you add a third and keep learning.

Yes, it was unlikely that *those* experienced nurses would make a mistake, but I wanted to be careful. When that first replacement set of nurses arrived, those with woefully limited skills, that habit became important. Mentored by a gifted nurse, I could stave off mistakes being made by less talented ones. Without that early mentoring, those children would have been in serious trouble.

Now I must explain something that may upset some. From what I could see, in an authoritarian system, the *more* talented a nurse is, the *more* likely she is to incur criticism from above. Indeed, in many cases it seemed attacks were most likely when nurses gave excellent care. Recall when nurses were attacked for helping that overloaded Hem-Onc nurse, or when I was criticized for giving excellent care to the teen boy who'd received cisplatin.

At first, that made no sense to me. I thought it was crazy. Why punish those who should be praised? Isn't criticism intended to improve care?

Not really. Remember the two new nurses I described who did so badly they had to repeat their orientation? As far as I know, their blunders didn't bring on them the wrath of the head nurse. After all, their poor orientation was as much her fault as my non-existent orientation had been. No, those nurses' problems had to continue long enough to be noticed higher up. Only then was action taken.

Yet when that second and more talented group of replacement nurses arrived there was almost immediate criticism aimed at them. Why was that? Because talented nurses make incompetent nurses look bad. That's why they are attacked, and why excellent care is treated as if it were a mistake.

That is bad and should never be allowed. When talented nurses get frustrated and leave, almost everyone loses. The only winners are the least capable nurses. Protecting talented nurses from the untalented is one role that a senior nurse mentor must play.

2. Capable Nurses

The second group of nurses are those of average ability, capable but not spectacular. There's nothing wrong with that. Mathematically, it's impossible for more than half a group to be above average. If hospitals hired only exceptional nurses, patients would die from a lack of care.

That's true in every area of life, including physicians. If anything, our residents, the product of four years of college *and* four years of medical school, made more serious mistakes than our nurses, who were the product of but two to four years of nursing school.

This means that most nurses will be good but not spectacular. Taught ten new things in class, they'll retain eight and discover a new one for themselves, for a total of nine. Is that terrible? No, like the CPR classes that we repeated each year, refresher courses will eventually teach a nurse all she needs to know. But those refresher courses must exist.

The critical difference between the exceptional and the capable nurse lies the necessity of offering on-going training for the latter. That training needs to be practical, dealing with common mistakes. It must remind nurses of what they were taught years before, such as reactions to vitamin K. Most important of all, it must deal with new issues that come up, such as central lines.

The third nurse in that second and more talented group of replacements was a capable nurse. I thought highly of her zeal to become professional. For her, skills were taught formally. She valued training and learned well from books and classes. That may be why she didn't grasp the risk of air embolism on her own. It wasn't being taught. She was the third nurse whose 'air in line' mistake I caught. Fortunately, in her case the air was still two feet shy of the patient. Other than the bother of forcing that air back through about six feet of tubing, no harm was done.

These different types of nurses respond differently to criticism. The exceptional are self-directed and far more critical of themselves than any head nurse could be. They know when they're being treated unfairly and respond objectively.

In contrast, capable nurses tend to be other-directed. Criticism from above is hard for them to handle. That's why I often thought of that third nurse as a 'nurse's nurse.' She worked hard because she wanted to be a good nurse by the standards of other nurses. Such nurses are dependent on others to teach them and rate them. When those others are overly critical, they take it badly.

That's precisely what happened to that third nurse one morning at change of shift. For some reason—probably teaching a CPR class—on that particular day I was late going home. When I dropped by Hem-Onc about 10 a.m., the head nurse pounced on me. Why, she asked, had I left a boy's sheets dirtied by stomach fluid from his suction line? I didn't know how to respond. The boy had been fine when I made my end-of-shift checks of each room.

That evening, I asked that nurse if she knew what had happened. She did. She had been in the room when I passed through. After I left, she moved the boy and some of his stomach juices squirted out a vent in his suction line onto the bed. That happened all the time and was no big deal. If she'd told me, I'd have changed his sheets. But she didn't, and I knew why. She was about to face criticism from those two crabby day nurses at morning report. She was in a panic and could think about nothing else.

I suggested that she might want to explain what actually happened to the head nurse, but I didn't push the matter. I felt sorry for what she had to face. I also knew that whatever criticism had been written up about me would remain in spite of evidence to the contrary. Fairness was rapidly disappearing from our unit. The head nurse hadn't bothered to investigate before she attacked me. She wouldn't bother to apologize or clear up my record afterward. Events like those were why nursing morale was collapsing and with it the quality of care for our children.

Nursing mistakes have several causes. Some result when a nurse simply fails to notice an error, perhaps in a medication order. The nurse has become so distracted, busy, tired or even relaxed, that she's inattentive. Other mistakes lie at the opposite extreme. An emergency occurs and a nurse panics, doing something stupid. Both kinds of mistakes can be countered by training. The first can be prevented by training nurses to remain alert and check what they do and the second by training them to respond calmly.

What we're discussing here is a third cause of nursing mistakes. You saw it in the incident I just mentioned. The nurse I was working with was not so inattentive that she failed to notice stomach fluid spilling onto the boy's sheets. Nor was that simple spill so scary that she did not know what to do. Telling me was obvious, yet she failed to do that because her mind was overwhelmed by a fear of criticism to come. Those nursing mistakes can be prevented by ending that culture of criticism.

3. *Failed Nurses*

Now we turn to the third group—those I call *failed nurses*. They're the ones who make it through school but fail at actual nursing. Their problem doesn't lie with insufficient teaching. It lies with a seeming inability to learn the actual practice of nursing. That's one reason they attach little value to training. It doesn't help them, so why should it help anyone else? What drives them is fear. That's why they think fear is so necessary.

Keep in mind that there's nothing wrong with not having a talent for nursing. Not everyone should be a nurse. The problem lies with those who aren't good at nursing but remain in the profession. Some of those who make it through nursing school should be encouraged to leave or at least move into areas where their inadequacies matter less. Processing paperwork or insurance claims is one option.

I can offer an illustration. I took readily to nursing care on Hem-Onc. From the very beginning, I felt like I belonged there and could handle its heavy emotional demands. I simply needed training. But I'm dreadful at foreign languages. No amount of linguistic training can alter that. I am stuck with English and can't learn another languages. When I've studied other languages, my teachers pitied me. I even pitied myself.

Fortunately, my incompetence at learning new languages does no one any harm. I'm not trying to make a living as a translator. Native speakers—and even many non-native ones—can spot my inability, so one is fooled, least of all me. I don't blame anyone but myself for my lack of talent, and I don't find fault with those who are good at languages.

Unfortunately, an inability in nursing is less obvious. Some people who can't nurse well often survive in the profession long enough to supervise those who do. That may explain many of the troubles I have described here. It is also why hospitals need senior nurse mentors who are exceptionally talented. The good can correct the bad.

Next we look at how the military has learned to deal with morale issues similar to those in nursing.

16. CHIEF OF THE BOAT

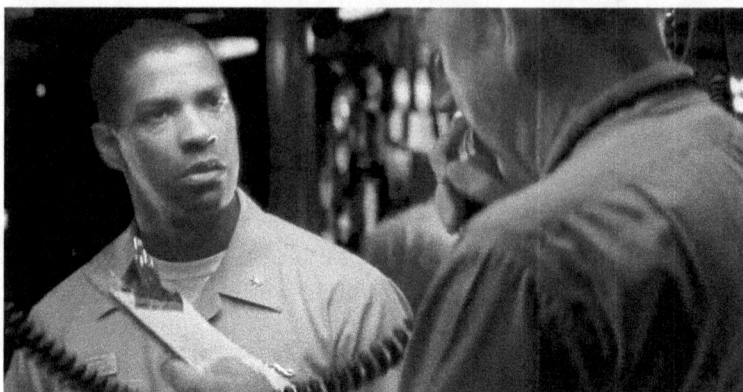

Initially, I wasn't sure whether I should include a marvelous leadership lesson that lies hidden in a scene from a popular movie. I feared that some might wonder what a film set on board a submarine equipped with nuclear missiles has to do with nursing care in a modern hospital. On the other hand, there are those who will understand that a staffing system that succeeds in the most trying of circumstances—an angry personal confrontation in which millions may die if the wrong choice is made—will also work in hospitals where life-or-death decisions take place on a much smaller scale.

Crimson Tide (1995) is set during the turmoil following the collapse of the Soviet Union. Rogue groups have taken over a military base equipped with nuclear missiles and are threatening to launch them against the United States and Japan. To counter that, the nuclear missile submarine *U.S.S. Alabama* has been dispatched to nearby waters. The movie's title comes from a nickname for the University of Alabama's football team, but also suggests the potential for bloodshed on an enormous scale.

The situation is tense. The only way to prevent the death of millions may be to preempt, launching a nuclear attack on the rebel base before it fires those missiles. In fact, the submarine receives orders to do just that, but the launch is delayed by a Russian attack submarine. In the process, the sub receives a partial second message. There's no way to know if the second message merely affirms the first or countermands it. That sets the stage for the film's climatic scene.

Knowing that even a few seconds delay might mean American cities get hit by nuclear missiles, the submarine's captain, played by Gene Hackman, wants to launch. He is opposed by his executive office (XO), played by Denzel Washington, who insists that they must get that second message in full before they act. He refuses to concur with captain's launch and, according to Navy regulations, no launch can take place without his concurrence.

Angry, the captain tells his executive officer, "You repeat this order, or I will find someone who will." The executive officer replies, "No, you won't sir," to which the Captain replies, "You are relieved of your position." He then calls out, "Cob, remove Mr. Hunter from the control room."

It's clear that what happens next—a preemptive nuclear attack or not—is up to this Cob. But who is he and why does he play such an important role? Why does the crew look to him to decide which of the two conflicting orders to obey?

At this point, many viewers miss something important. Some may even think that the person on which the Captain was calling was named Cob. Not true, Cob is a position rather a name. It stands for "COB" or Chief of the Boat. He's the senior non-commissioned, enlisted member of a U.S. Navy submarine. Senior as in a senior nursing mentor.

In the U.S. Navy, a COB plays a key role in the relationship between a submarine's commanding officers and its crew. He reports directly to the Captain and Executive Officer and advises them about conditions involving the crew. He is also responsible for the daily running of the submarine and for the discipline of the crew.

That's why the film's scriptwriters got it right. The COB was precisely the person to decide which of those conflicting orders were to be obeyed. In the film, his response is, "Captain, please, the XO is right. You can't launch unless he concurs." Despite his anger, the Captain knew the crew would follow the COB and not him.

A short time later, they get the full version of that second message. The Russian rebels have been defeated. There is no longer a danger of a nuclear attack, and the sub is ordered to stand down.

How did that scene appear in this book? When I mentioned what I was writing in an email to a nephew who is a Navy doctor, he replied, "Sounds like a Command Master Chief role." When I reminded him that I know little about the Navy, he emailed back:

> The command master chief is the highest ranking enlisted member at a command; they report directly and only to the commanding officer. The army, air force and marine corps all have a similar structure with different names. They monitor and advocate for enlisted members of the command, ensure morale and discipline, etc.

After doing research of my own, I discovered that on a Navy submarine that position is called Chief of the Boat or COB. At that point, I recalled the scene from *Crimson Tide* and saw its relevance.

Of course, there are major differences between a submarine and a hospital. What works with one may not work with the other. I'm certainly *not* suggesting that a senior nurse mentor should replace the nursing administration in the day-to-day management of nursing staff like a COB manages the day-to-day running of a submarine. In fact, the value of her position may be that she's *not* caught up in the conflicts of interest that would create.

No, what I am suggesting is that some nursing administrations may fail to "effective monitor and advocate for" the nursing staff. They might act like the "bad cop" in police questioning without having someone take on the role of the "good cop." That results in a failure of "morale and discipline" much like it would on a submarine. That's because wearing two hats is difficult. A nursing administration focused on after-the-fact fault-finding and blame-placing will often fail to provide encouragement for nurses to do their job well.

One strength of a senior nurse mentor flows from the fact that she's not caught up in fixing blame or in appeasing administrators obsessed with costs. She can keep her focus on nurses, their morale, and how well prepared they are for their responsibilities. Much like similar positions in the military, she reports "directly and only" to the hospital's CEO. Only the CEO can discipline or fire her.

A senior nurse mentor is also spared time-consuming distractions. She does not run well-established training programs such as

CPR. Those remain under the nursing administration. But she can make up for short-term deficiencies in those programs.

That includes one deficiency often missed by hospitals. A nurse who *almost* makes a mistake, but catches it at the last moment, can talk with a senior nurse mentor, knowing that what she says won't go into her personnel file. The nurse can say: "There's a problem with this new procedure that you might want to make sure other nurses know about before something bad happens." That's better than what often happens today, where trouble-avoidance waits for something bad to actually happen. The result is often a costly lawsuit.

For instance, with the central line example I use in this book, the senior nurse mentor might get the surgery department to tell her the names of every patient getting a central line. Then she could go to those patients' nurses, asking: "Are you trained in central lines?" If not, she'll make sure those nurse get the proper training without being graded down for not knowing what they've not been taught.

In short, a senior nurse mentor would operate *alongside* the nursing administration while not being a part of it. She could talk with anyone and exert her influence everywhere while reporting directly only to the CEO. Her work would *complement* that of the nursing administration, doing what it cannot do. In practice, they should love her, since she'll be taking responsibilities off their shoulders and preventing costly mistakes.

Interestingly, while the various branches of the U.S. military have long had those responsible for morale, the *formal* role of Command Master Chief (and thus the COB) is quite recent, only being established about 1995. A Wikipedia article has this to say in the formal language of the Navy.

First referenced in OPNAVINST 1306.2C dated 16 October 1995 (now 1036.2G), the Navy's command master chief program is intended to stimulate free-flowing communications, and ensure the highest standards of professionalism are upheld at all levels within the chain of command. Command master chiefs strengthen the chain of command by keeping the commanding officer aware of existing or potential situations as well as procedures and practices which affect the mission, readiness, welfare and morale of the sailors in the command.

CMCs are the senior enlisted leaders who report directly to their respective commanding officers. They formulate and implement policies concerning morale, welfare, job satisfaction, discipline, utilization and training of navy personnel. By reporting directly to their commanding officer, the CMCs keep their chain of command aware and informed of sensitive and current issues.

My brother in law, who was in the U.S. Army, told me another indication of just how important these positions are considered by the military. A commanding officer who wants to talk to a command master chief can't simply order a conversation. He must *request* permission to speak, an indication of the high honor and responsibility attached to the position. **A senior nurse mentor should be accorded similar respect. She's not to be bossed around, certainly not by the nursing administration and not even by the hospital's CEO.**

Now for an important question. Should nursing imitate the U.S. military? Certainly not. But there is enough similarity between the two that nursing can learn helpful lessons about maintaining morale and retaining expensively trained staff from the military. The military made those formal changes in the 1990s to deal with an all-voluntary military. Hospitals need to take similar measures to deal with high nursing turnover. Even a modest reduction in that turnover would more than cover a senior nurse mentor's salary.

In the next chapter, we look at psychological factors that complicate giving good nursing care, particularly under the stress that harsh criticism creates.

17. Loyalty and Focus

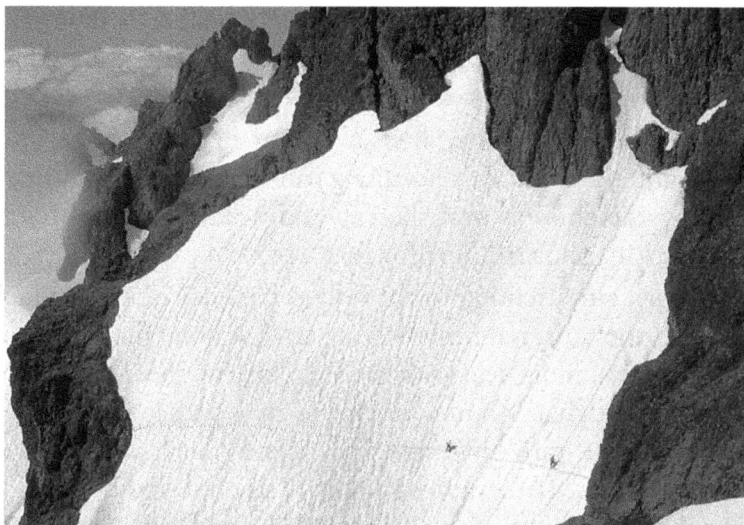

In this chapter, we continue to look at how problems are handled in high-stress situations within other fields to better understand how to deal with similar situations in hospitals. Later we'll look at how business deals with troublesome issues.

Although I've forgotten the specifics, the scene is one of my favorites. Long ago, probably in Africa, a patch of newly exposed clay was rendered soft by a rain that fell in the night and had not yet been baked hard by the mid-day sun. Perhaps it was 100,000 years ago, perhaps more. That mud, baked rock-hard, remains to this day.

In that drying mud we see three sets of footprints of differing sizes. The largest are almost certainly those of a man and the smaller of a woman. Between them are the tiny footprints of a child. Think of a father and mother, with the child walking between them and holding on to a hand of each. The child, who in my retelling is a little girl, senses danger and grips all the more tightly.

In my imagination, I see that long-ago family traveling a little further and crossing a meadow with grass so high it reaches to the mother's shoulders. Suddenly out of the grass perhaps 20 yards in front of them, an adult male lion rears up. It's hungry and sees them as prey. Their only chance at safety is a tall tree over a hundred yards away through a dense thicket of briers and brambles.

What happens next matters because I believe it represents the essence of what being truly human means. What those two parents do is what we as humans should do.

We notice the mother first. Without hesitation, she grabs up her daughter and plunges headlong into those briers and brambles, shielding the child as best she can and heedless of the thorns ripping her skin. She's running for that tree.

We turn our attention to the father. He's not moved an inch. He stands all the taller, communicating to that lion, "Before you get to my family, you must deal with me." Perhaps by sheer force of will he can intimidate that lion into moving away—perhaps not. To prepare for the latter, he raises high his stone-tipped club and focuses on the danger he faces. If the lion attacks, he has but one hope. He must bring that club down with all his strength and with perfect timing. The tip of the stone must come down at the center of the lion's forehead in a terrific killing blow. No other strike will succeed.

That long-ago scene fades away. The point I wanted to make has been made. It has revealed two of the traits that help define our humanity. They are *loyalty*, which we might also call love, and *focus*.

The father and mother demonstrate *loyalty* to one another and the child they love. The mother knows the father will stand and fight that lion even at the cost of his life. The father knows the mother will do her best to get their child to safety. Even the child, young as she is, knows to trust them. That's why she gripped their hands.

At this point, we should not become shrill or ideological. It's pointless to claim that the father or mother is braver. The mother risks her life fleeing with her daughter rather than without. The father risks his life by standing up to the lion. The difference does not lie in their bravery, but how they demonstrate their love. Each does what he or she does best. The stronger fights the lion, the other tends the child. That may be why under stress men tend to a fight-or-flight response, while women tilt toward tend-or-befriend.

The other trait you see is *focus*. In the presence of so much danger, both the mother and father must focus on what matters and ignore all else. The mother must run with every ounce of her strength and ignore the thorns ripping at her skin. The father must set aside any fear he feels, project more confidence than he actually possesses, and stand fast when the lion attacks. Flight at that point is folly. His only hope lies in a well-struck blow. On that he must put his all.

That long-ago story matters because it illustrates the deeply held attitudes that people often display in a crisis. And yes, I am aware that not everyone responds that way. Some are cowards and blame-shifters. I write about them here too.

An experience I had while mountain climbing also illustrates loyalty and focus. If you're ever in Seattle, look west across Puget Sound toward the Olympic mountains. The largest mountain you'll see is Mount Constance, rising almost 7,800 feet above the water. Starting at a low elevation, it takes many hours to summit and return. In the case of my climbing partner and I, that meant about 16 hours on the move without a rest. That came on top of having almost no sleep the night before.

We took a standard route to the top. On the mountain's upper slopes we came to snowfield called the Terrible Traverse. That's it pictured at the start of this chapter. Notice the two tiny climbers. They're another party taking the same route years earlier. Scary isn't it? Mountain climbing can be like that. It's not for the faint of heart.

Why is that crossing so terrible? Because many snow fields are gentle. They level out at the bottom, so those who slip come to a gradual stop. This one is a killer. It's not only extremely steep, as you can see, it also ends in giant boulders. A climber who slips may be killed outright or die before help arrives.

We reached the Terrible Traverse in early afternoon. We roped up and began putting on our crampons. That's a steel frame with sharp spikes that clamps to boots and is used for walking or climbing on snow and ice.

The guy I was with finished first and started across. He'd only taken a single step when I heard a yell and saw him began to plummet down that steep slope. In a little over two seconds, the 50-foot rope that joined us would snap taunt. A series of images flashed though my mind too quickly for words.

First, I saw myself as I was on that bare rock with no hand holds to grab. When that rope ran out, I imagined myself snatched away, sending both of us plummeting to our deaths.

Second, a solution came from deep inside. I saw myself grabbing the remaining rope still coiled on the rock and exerting as much drag with my hands as possible. That might save our lives.

Third, came a disturbing image. It showed what might happen as that rope burned through my hands. I saw them ripped apart, with bones and muscles exposed. I grabbed anyway. Anything was better than that terrible plunge.

Whether my hands offered enough resistance or not, I'll never know, but when the rope snapped taunt, I remained on the rock. My friend twisted around and slammed into the rocks on the side of the snowfield, but was otherwise unhurt. I looked down at my hands and was surprised to see them merely reddened from friction.

Our lesson learned, we abandoned the Terrible Traverse, climbed down the rocks on one side, crossed at the bottom, and climbed back up to the route on the other side. We reached the summit and returned by a different route.

You see in that climbing incident the same traits as in that long-ago tale. Both loyalty and focus were present. Displaying *loyalty*, I didn't release that rope, which was only attached to a nylon web around my waist by a quick-release carabiner. Displaying *focus* on what mattered, I was willing to see my hands ripped to shreds.

Traits like those are not just for life-threatening situations. They can appear in stressful situations in a hospital as easily as on a mountain. But they come with a serious downside. In more complex situations, that instinctive stress on loyalty and focus can keep us from thinking clearly or seeing all we should see. That matters a lot.

No, I'm not arguing that loyalty and focus meant I decided badly in the crises I faced at the hospital. I believe I did well. No child died because of a mistake of mine, nor did any child suffer harmful consequences from a bad choice I made. My loyalty to them did that. I also did not betray the nurses I was working with even under pressure from cranky head nurses. I did what mattered. Loyalty and focus were why.

On Hem-Onc I was right to give those children my first loyalty and to avoid, as much as possible, that war between nurses. Those ill-tempered day nurses could have crippled my ability to care for those kids. On the teen unit, I was right to refuse to give the head nurse any criticism of nurses. They were under enough pressure.

Perhaps I was also right, given what little I knew, not to raise a fuss about training. That I will never know. There were too many unknowns in how the administration might respond, particularly given that what I'd be saying was an implicit criticism of their decisions. I couldn't put at risk my ability to care for those children. By that point I had several times more experience in their care than the on-duty resident and *all* the nurses I was working with *combined.* Those children needed my watchful eyes.

No, as I look back, what frustrated me weren't the choices I made. Given what I knew at the time, I did the best I could. **The problem lay in how my stress-induced loyalty and focus limited my ability to *imagine* other and more creative solutions that might have reconciled the conflicts I felt. Perhaps the choices I felt were necessary really weren't.**

Recall those illustrations and you'll see what I mean. That long-ago father had only two choices. He could stand up to the lion or he could run away. Those were his *only* options. Loyalty meant he stayed to protect his family. Focus gave him the best chance of coming out alive. That was good.

In my climbing experience, there were again two options. I could disconnect the rope that joined me to my friend, or I could do my best to arrest his plunge. Those were the *only* solutions. Again, loyalty and focus drove my actions and were useful. I couldn't waste time looking for alternatives because there were none.

At the hospital, although *my* life was never in danger, the lives of the children I was caring for were. That created stresses not that different from those in a wilderness. The choices I made mattered for them, and my thinking was shaped by stress.

Now look at the choices I *felt* I faced. Should I focus on children or on training policies? I was responsible for those children and owed them my loyalty. I wasn't responsible for training. But notice how complex my choices were. This wasn't run or stand. This was taking a stand in two areas that *seemed* to conflict.

If I had displayed more imagination, the problem of central line training actually had a solution. Yes, I knew approaching the head nurse was futile, while approaching the nursing administration was risky. But there was someone who not only had a strong interest in seeing that central lines were safe, he had the authority to say, "This *will* be taught." That was the line's inventor, one of our most respected physicians. My work in Hem-Onc was enough to get me a meeting with him. Why didn't I think of that? Alas, as I have been saying, intense loyalty and focus narrowed my thinking. I couldn't see any solution other than those directly in front of me.

Look at my other problem. Should my focus lie on my young patients or with those much put-upon nurses? Again, I chose the children. The dangers they faced were far greater. But might I have helped both?

Later, I realized that I had another option. I did not have to take on those day nurses in a battle royal and risk their ire and that of the head nurse. I could suggest to the night nurses that they complain as a group to the director of nursing. That would not have involved me directly and might have gotten results.

Recall I told you that engineer's adage, "When you're up to your neck in alligators, it's hard to remember that your original goal was to drain the swamp." What I've described here is like that, but rather than forget our *goals* under pressure, we lose our ability to come up with *solutions*. That's why, when we recall a problem later, we often ask ourselves why we didn't think of seemingly obvious answers. During my time at the hospital, there were several situations I faced whose solution only came to me later. That's frustrating.

There is a reason why, under stress, our minds often become less imaginative. In many dangerous situations, debate can result in dangerous delays. Remember what I said about the Incident Command and the importance of deciding quickly? Our minds often function as an ICS whose goal is to reduce our choices to a manageable size. It knows an obvious decision made quickly is often better than a less obvious but better one made too late.

But many hospital situations do not require a split-second response. More complicated responses are needed, ones that require reflection and thought. That makes them harder to see. Here's an example where only seeming luck saved me.

One night we were finishing up chemotherapy on a two-year-old girl, the Wendy of *My Nights* that I mentioned in Chapter 12. We hadn't been able to complete her chemotherapy in the alloted 24-hours, so the resident ordered a two-hour extension. That often happened. Then he and the nurse left, while the girl's mother took a much-needed break. I was left with a little girl who was oblivious to all that was happening.

Within seconds, a nagging thought came to me. On an earlier visit, Wendy screamed when anyone but her mother approached. Now she seemed unaware that her mother had left or that I was holding her. "Not good," I thought, "something is wrong." In a flash, I hit the call button. The nurse, knowing it was me, would come quickly. Then I realized that I faced a problem. Other than my gut-level feeling, I could offer no reason for ending Wendy's chemotherapy. What was I going to say to persuade both nurse and resident to reverse a decision made only moments before?

A few seconds later one of Wendy's feet twitched. I knew what that meant. I had her on her side in bed and was gently restraining her when a *grand mal* seizure hit. No further explanation was needed. Her chemotherapy was stopped, and shortly after that she was transferred to the ICU.

Notice the difficulties I faced. This wasn't me reacting to a hungry lion or a falling climber. I wasn't even in charge of the response. I needed reasons that would persuade others. That made matters far more complicated. But for that fortuitous seizure, I don't know what I would have done.

That's a major problem in hospitals. Stresses, many of them unnecessarily created by the administration or other staff, make it hard to think clearly and creatively precisely when such thinking is need most. That can be frustrating. What can help find answers?

Training can help. Those whose work is dangerous train constantly. That's why on the teen unit, I knew how to handle that girl's air embolism and her nurse didn't. I'd thought and trained myself to be ready. In an emergency, hesitation can be fatal, so you need to prepare. Emergency workers often refer to situations where "their training kicked in." That's what they mean. Their response is decisive and unhesitatingly quick.

Even when training fails to offer a specific answer, having similar training can help. When you've trained well, the presence of an unexpected situation is less likely to cause you to freeze. Before my Mount Constance climb, I'd practiced arrests on glaciers, where the proper respond to a partner slipping was to go into an arrest position, lying face down in the snow and holding tightly to an ice axe thrust deeply into the glacier. I couldn't do that on bare rock, but my mind remained calm and found an alternative. Even when training doesn't have a specific answer to your problem, it can give you the confidence to discover the right one.

When a problem is outside the scope of training, broader knowledge can help. The account of "Oblivious Brian" in *My Nights* is an example. No amount of training based on what was known at that time could have prepared me for dealing with his situation and yet I did. I leveraged what I knew to find an answer that wasn't even in the leukemia protocols.

Here's what happened. About two a.m., as Brian was finishing up his initial chemotherapy, I became worried. He'd been admitted with a platelet count lower than most newly diagnosed patients. That led to a nose bleed that the usual remedies did not fix, so a resident was packing the boy's nose with gauze. As he did, a nagging idea popped into my mind. "That has to be painful," I thought, "and yet he is showing no reaction."

I searched through all I knew. Low platelets wouldn't cause that oblivion nor would chemotherapy on its own. Yet the timing mattered. There had to be something wrong. But what?

I knew the resident had ordered a CBC, a complete blood count, to monitor those low platelets. Because leukemia is a cancer of the blood, I knew that one more test, a blood chemistry, would provide an overview of Brian's situation. Perhaps the answer lay there.

I stopped the resident as he left and suggested that, since the boy had been vomiting, it might be a good idea to run a blood chemistry. Yes, I knew that was bosh, that his vomiting had not been enough for that. But some instinct said Brian's problem might show up in his blood chemistry. Any reason, however dubious, that would get the resident to order that test was worth mentioning. He agreed and added an order for a blood chemistry.

Just after I left work, that lab result came back with all alarms ringing. Brian's blood chemistry was so far off, he was rushed to the ICU. Fortunately, his problem was caught early enough that he was back on Hem-Onc that evening.

That was early Monday morning. At report on Thursday, the evening nurse had news. The reason for Brian's emergency had been discovered and the national leukemia protocol altered to prevent it from happening again. He had tumor lysis syndrome.

In the wee hours of Monday morning, I'd displayed a remarkable characteristic of the human mind—our amazing ability to intuit answers without fully understanding why. I'd come up with the answer to a problem whose existence wasn't even known at the time.

No, I hadn't found the cause of Brian's troubles. Remember my limited training. I didn't even know what normal blood chemistry values are and had never heard of tumor lysis syndrome. But I did know kids being treated for leukemia. I patched together enough from that to start a process that did find answers. You don't have to know *everything* to know *enough*. Never forget that.

Finally, every answer that I've described thus far faces a serious problem. All hinge on the abilities of an individual nurse. Training requires that she be trained, as does extending that training into new areas. Even an ability to act beyond training takes time to develop. My response to Brian's condition was a result of spending perhaps two-thousand hours caring for children with leukemia and thinking about them constantly. That is why I instinctively knew something was wrong with him. If I had been recently hired, I would not have known that.

That's also why, when training and experience come up short, there needs to be more resources available. I'm sure you've guessed what that is. It's the opportunity to consult with someone who is not only better trained and more experienced, but also emotionally removed from those imagination-restricting stresses. Such a person can see answers that those closer to a problem may not see. She can help clarify those vague, nagging doubts.

Physicians have such a person. It's common in medicine to call in another physician when the patient is a member of one's own family. Why? Because doctors know from bitter experience that, when one's own child is involved, their judgment can be seriously flawed. A much-loved son may be showing signs of leukemia. Yet, blinded by love, his dad may to fail to see that. Doctors need another doctor to see what they are unable to see.

Nurses are no different. They can grow so attached to patients or torn by the stresses at work, that a blindness creeps in. The answer lies the nursing equivalent of a physician calling on a colleague. Most of the time, that's another nurse, typically one with more experience. But sometimes it might be a senior nurse mentor.

Next, we look at a mysterious visitor Hem-Onc had shortly after I starting working there and the secret she revealed.

18. MYSTERIOUS VISITOR

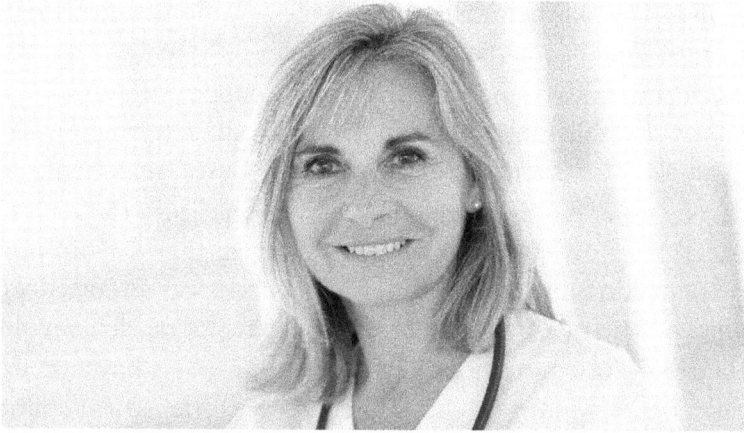

To my later regret, I didn't keep a diary of what I've been describing here. All I have are vivid memories of certain events that contain clues as to their dating. I almost always remember the patient's room and a sense of the season. Hem-Onc could get chilly in the winter, and the sun rose much earlier in the summer. That helps. The nurse I was working with offers another clue. One experience often informed another, so that establishes their order. Most helpful of all is the feeling the surrounds an event. My last months on Hem-Onc came with a haunting fear that the clash between nurses meant danger for our kids. That colored everything.

Coloring is how I know the incident with a mysterious visitor came early, perhaps during my first month on Hem-Onc. What I was doing was still so new, a nurse that I'd never seen before showing up in the wee hours of the night did not strike me as unusual. Later, I would have been more curious about who she was.

She was in her forties and thus older than most. The hospital liked to hire young, so the typical floor nurse was in her twenties, while most specialty nurses were in their thirties. She may have worked in an out-patient clinic. Since she had come to Hem-Onc, it might have been the leukemia clinic. Checking on me—new on nights—may have even been one reason for her visit. She certainly went out of her way to talk with me.

She did more than chat. She confided something surprising. The hospital, she said, had a history of going off on a tangent about every five years. The last time had been about three years earlier when its specialists decided their colleagues in the community didn't need to be kept informed about patients they'd referred.

It's easy to understand why that might happen. These specialists were busy. Establishing phone contact with the referring physicians was a hassle. They felt it was better to stay focused on patient care.

On the other hand, the referring physicians knew those children remained their patients and, when discharged, they'd again provide care. They didn't like feeling that when a child was admitted a door slammed in their face with an implied "you're not needed anymore."

The result, my mysterious visitor went on, was a boycott. When possible, doctors sent sick children elsewhere. The patient count fell so low, she said, some units had to be closed. It was grim.

I had no reason to doubt her, and a few months later I received confirmation. Rummaging in a nursing-station drawer I came across a motivational lapel pin whose slogan was along the lines of "Have You Talked to the Referring?" The hospital had learned a lesson.

During my last, troubled months at work, I recalled that mysterious visitor and her 'every five years' warning. Three years before, she had said, and now it was roughly two years later. Her prediction was disturbingly accurate.

Another thought troubled me. On Hem-Onc, I had tried to explain the tensions between nurses as the envy that older, untalented nurses had for younger, prettier, and more capable nurses. That was less disturbing than the possibility that those destructive attitudes originated higher up.

There's much to be said for that. In *The Sociopath Next Door*, Martha Stout writes of an all-too-common *covetous sociopath*, "Since it is simply not possible to steal and have for oneself the most valuable 'possessions' of another person—beauty, intelligence, success, a strong character—the covetous sociopath settles for besmirching or damaging enviable qualities in others so they will not have them, either, or at least not be able to enjoy them so much."

Unfortunately, that explanation did not work on the teen unit, at least not among the nurses. All its nurses were attractive, capable and got along well. Instead, the problems only began *after* the permanent head nurse returned. As she attempted to set nurse against nurse, morale plummeted. I came to suspect that, whatever their own internal motivations were, these trouble-making head nurses were also responding to pressures from the administration.

At this point, some disclaimers are needed. First, when I started work I saw nothing, apart from those poor orientations given to me and the nurses hired a few months after me, that indicated serious trouble ahead. All seemed well. In fact, I saw the opposite. I was impressed by the responsibilities the hospital gave me. I was soon teaching CPR and monitoring peritoneal dialysis.

The latter was with an incredibly primitive machine. Since Seattle hospitals pioneered kidney dialysis, nurses joked that it was "pediatric peritoneal dialysis machine number one." Perhaps that was true. Online, I found a picture of one that looked similar. It had been hand-built at a nearby hospital in 1964.

The nursing administration must have trusted me because, other than my vigilance, that clumsy collection of large glass bottles, industrial timers, rubber hoses, and clanking valves had no safety features. The machine had lingered on far beyond its time for one reason. When a child had a peritoneal tube surgically implanted, it provided their first overnight test of whether dialysis would be tolerated. That didn't happen often enough to justify buying a state-of-the-art machine.

My second disclaimer stresses that not all units were equally affected. I've already mentioned that the teen unit was fine when I transferred there. That was thanks to a sweet temporary head nurse. She was wonderful. Nothing could make her mean-spirited.

I was also impressed with the spirit of the nurses when I floated to Babyland, the unit that cared for most children under one. The joy they displayed was so great, I envied them. Impressed by what I saw of their head nurse, she's one role model for a senior nurse mentor. She motivated and taught rather than criticized and blamed.

My final disclaimer concerns that five-year cycle. I have no reason to believe that the cycle continue beyond the troubles that immediately followed my departure. **Keep in mind that I am not singling out *any* hospital in this book. As many nurses will point out, my**

experience is hardly unique. Mistakes like those I describe could happen in almost any hospital. That's why I wrote this book and why a senior nurse mentor is so important.

Necessity now forces me to explore a topic about which my knowledge is limited. I've already mentioned meeting the hospital's head of nursing in an interview three months after I started. She told me my EMT training had gotten me that Hem-Onc position. I had the impression she was happy with the result, which was reassuring because she seemed to be a stern disciplinarian.

Strange as it sounds, I had more contact with the CEO than with her. Every so often, our CPR team would meet at 8 a.m. in a conference room next to the cafeteria. Since I finished on Hem-Onc by 7:30, the person in charge had asked me to show up early and make sure the room was properly set up.

Conference rooms were scheduled by the hour and the previous user was supposed to leave ten minutes before the hour. I showed up about five minutes before and found the room still occupied by none other than the CEO and two others. The result was not happy.

Yes, I probably should have been apologetic with the guy who was my ultimate boss. But like many who work nights, I attached a high value to the sleep I was missing thanks to this pesky meeting. By missing sleep to teach CPR, I felt that I was doing the hospital a favor. I wasn't feeling meek.

We exchanged a few words that avoided the real issue—that he should have been gone already. Later, when I thought about it, I concluded that nothing would happen. He was so many levels above me that he'd look silly trying to get even.

I need not worry. I ran into him in a hallway a few weeks later. He remembered me and seemed eager to be friendly. I concluded that, while anyone in his position would have to be good at bureaucratic gamesmanship, he could be trusted to play fair.

Unfortunately, none of those contacts, brief as they were, explain why relations between the administration and nurses turned so sour. Neither struck me as warm and emphatic. But both seemed capable, with none of the mean-spirited, blame-placing attitude I saw in some head nurses. Where personalities were involved, I have no answers.

I did develop an explanation for those troubles while studying medical ethics at the University of Washington and learning about recent events in medicine. What I concluded hinged on two then-recent changes in hospital care that placed administrators between the proverbial rock and a hard place.

The rock was a change in how the government reimbursed medical costs that began under the Carter administration and was called Diagnostic Related Groups (DRGs). Instead of paying *all the costs* associated with a particular patient, the government would pay a *fixed amount* based on a patient's diagnosis.

For acute appendicitis, for instance, there'd be a determined-in-advance payment. A hospital that handled such a patient well and discharged them early would make a modest profit. If complications developed, the hospital would absorb the added costs. Policy makers—obsessed as ever with their schemes—believed DRGs would force hospitals to control costs and didn't consider that the change might have other effects. At that time, DRGs were *not* being applied to pediatric care, but administrators at a children's hospital had good reason to suspect that would come.

The hard place was a rapid increase in malpractice costs. Tort lawyers had found ways around the traditional legal protections extended to non-profits and were greedily grabbing their 40 percent slice of huge settlements. I forget the exact figures, but recall that they were astonishing. Over the space of about eight years, the cost of hospital malpractice insurance increased roughly 600 percent. If you were a hospital administrator, that was most unsettling.

Worst of all, those two changes worked against one another. DRGs pressured hospitals to take shortcuts to reduce costs, running fewer tests and discharging patients earlier. In contrast, lawsuits pressured hospitals to practice defensive medicine, running more tests and doing more expensive procedures than normal to reduce risks and appear better in court.

Now recall what I've written about stress causing people to narrow their loyalties and limit their focus. As the stress on the administration grew, did their loyalties narrow and their focus became more restricted? If so, who were the chief losers?

I suspect they were the dedicated nurses I worked with. Their wages were one of the hospital's largest expenses. That helps explain the growing pressure that Hem-Onc nurses complained about, as well as the too-heavy workload on the teen day shift.

Still worse, many lawsuits could be blamed, rightly or wrongly, on nursing errors. Nurses were easier to blame than the physicians, particularly the senior specialists who brought in the money. In a blame-shifting culture, actual guilt matters less than the ease with which a group can be blamed.

Nurses are easy to blame. Take that order for vitamin K via IV that I mentioned earlier. The nurse I was working with questioned the order's good sense. The girl had been taking that vitamin by pill for years with no ill-effects. Why suddenly change to something known to be more risky?

She was right, and fortunately she was smart enough prepare for the reaction which followed. But what if she'd been less skilled? My hunch is that a physician's stupid order would *not* result in discipline, but a nurse's clumsy response would. That's not fair.

I suspect that may be how blaming nurses began and why it grew so terrible. In my last few months at the hospital the head nurse was threatening to fire nurses who did not change. As a motivational technique, that's astonishingly stupid.

A blame culture like that results in the two problems that we have already discussed. First, under criticism, nurses make *more* mistakes rather than less. Second, fearful of what might happen, nurses turn silent and their frustrations don't reach administrators. Seeing no hope for change, their only option is to quit.

That was certainly true then. My resignation letter and the remarks I made about overwork were the only open complaints I heard about. Since I was leaving, writing that letter was easy, and since I wasn't a career nurse, I had nothing to lose. While I didn't directly attack the head nurse, I didn't need to do so. The fact that she'd not discovered just how overworked those nurses were condemned her by implication. When the two of us met for one last time, she was most unhappy with me, but I didn't care. She had inflicted so much misery on nurses I liked, I wasn't sad to see her suffer painful consequences.

There was one exception to that no complaining rule, although it came only a month or so before I left and didn't involve nurses. Two new nursing assistants had been hired with the understanding that they'd constitute one full-time position on the teen unit. Both were mothers of small children who wanted to be able to stay home when their child was sick. They agreed among themselves to an informal flex-time. When A's child was sick, B would fill in and vice-versa.

I saw that as marvelous, particularly since both were much better suited to day's busy-but-dull bustle than I was. As mothers, they wanted work that wasn't emotionally exhausting. With fewer outside responsibilities, I preferred high-stress accompanied by greater accomplishment. For me, day shift on the teen unit was filled with drudgery. Only the joy I got from knowing patients and seeing them get well kept me from quitting sooner.

Unfortunately, the hospital reneged on its agreement and required both women to work full-time. That suggests that turnover was high even among assistants and that a staffing crisis was already quietly developing. I do know that almost none of the assistants that I had oriented with two years earlier were still at the hospital.

To their credit, those two women openly complained, as least to others on the unit. If the administration had been more willing to listen to complaints such as theirs, it might have avoided the crisis to come. Unfortunately, it did not.

These growing tensions would have also corrected themselves if there'd been a senior nurse mentor immune to administrative pressure and in a position to speak up. She could talk with the nursing staff, hear their complaints, investigate them, and then turn around to confront the administration with the frustrations that nurses were afraid to discuss openly.

Next, we turn to the business world. One of the world's largest corporations has an intriguing, high-level position dedicated to solving financial, morale and staffing problems much like those that can develop in hospitals. That's next.

19. RESPONDING TO TROUBLE

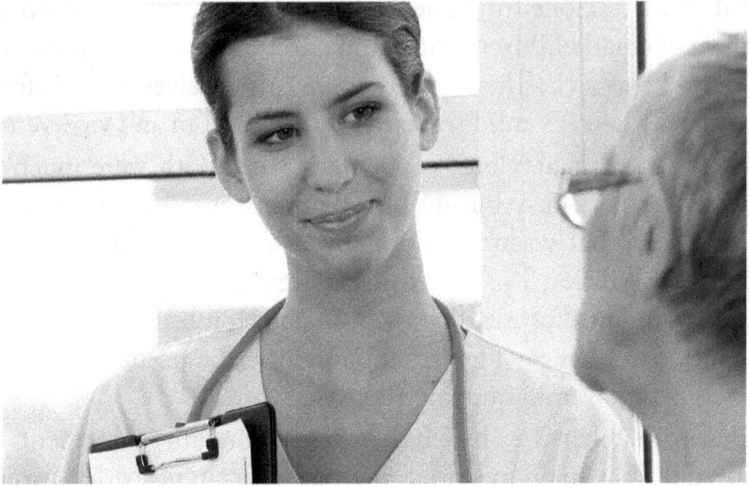

Variety has been the spice of my life. A few years after working at that children's hospital, I found myself in yet another field, first as a technical proofreader for Microsoft and later as a technical writer for Boeing.

Boeing is one of the world's largest businesses, manufacturing about half the world's commercial aircraft, as well as managing a host of other highly complex projects fraught with risk. Make a mistake designing a new aircraft, and the cost overruns could run into the billions. Make other mistakes, and hundreds of people might die. It's not a fault-tolerant environment.

So how does Boeing handle those risks? A friend gave me a unique insight. His father held a position so high up in the company that his boss reported to the CEO of Boeing. That's high.

If you imagine Boeing's corporate chart, there'd be a CEO at the top. Underneath him would be the heads of the company's major divisions, such as Boeing Commercial, Boeing Military, and Boeing Corporate. Each by itself would be one of the largest businesses on the planet. Beneath each division would be the company's major projects. Under Boeing Commercial, for instance, might be a division building the 787 aircraft. That's the level where my friend's father worked. He ranked equal to those who managed budgets in the billions and had thousand of employees under them. Yet he had a modest budget and typically only six people reporting to him.

What did he do that was so important to rank that high? For one thing, his team set the high-level computer security standards for the entire company. A failure there could lead to disaster, especially with secretive 'black hole' military projects. But he also played another critical role. When a serious problem arose, say the development of a new aircraft fell behind schedule, his team would be brought in to discover what had gone wrong.

Operating under the direct orders of the CEO, he had the authority to look into anything and question anyone. That explains his high rank. He stood equal to or higher than anyone he might be investigating. Since he stood outside the design or production divisions, he would never be investigating his boss. Most important of all, he'd advanced so far, he would never be tempted to further his career by covering something up. That matters.

The result was, as he once told me, he investigated objectively and let the chips fall where they may. He was unimpeachable. His job was to get the facts, report them, and recommend action. He was perfect for that job—fair, honest, and no nonsense.

Do *hospitals* need someone in precisely that role? Not really. They are far smaller than Boeing. In similar situations they should probably hire outside consultants. But *hospital nursing* does need someone who plays a similarly independent role, someone who is as far outside the hospital's normal structure as my friend's dad was at Boeing. That is because every organization needs an independent check on failure. Without that, mistakes are almost certain to happen. With that check, they either don't happen or get soon corrected.

In this book, I call those who provide an in-house check on nursing failures senior nurse mentors, enlarging on an existing role rather than inventing a new one. That's because there are similarities between a traditional mentor and a senior nurse mentor.

Here's a description of a nurse mentor from KC Health Careers. I've adapted it by turning their major points into a bulleted list.

- Mentoring may be a formal or informal process that works best when it is intentional.
- The purpose of mentoring is to encourage, support and guide nurses in their positions, so that they will continue to grow personally and professionally.
- Mentors are coaches, advisors, friends, cheerleaders and counselors.
- Mentors are not responsible for the nurse's day-to-day activities or for solving problems.
- Mentors do not evaluate the mentee and should have no direct link to the mentee's supervisor.
- Mentors generally do not teach specific position-related skills or tasks.
- Mentors offer a nonjudgmental listening ear for the mentee.
- Depending on what the mentee needs and desires, the mentor may help with continued socialization within the institution, communication issues, career goals and problem solving.
- Through their own experiences and expertise, mentors can help the mentee determine what steps to take and appropriate resources.
- The mentoring relationship is built on trust and is confidential.
- A formal mentoring relationship is usually time limited and ranges anywhere from six months to a year. However, some mentoring relationships become life-long.

That's almost, but not quite, what this book suggests. The senior nurse mentors I describe are experienced nurses involved in solving *some* problems, particularly those involving morale and short-term training. Think of them as freelance troubleshooters. If there's an issue, they can operate independently, much like my friend's dad did when he investigated Boeing's woes.

There are other differences. That list allows a nurse mentor to have additional responsibilities that might limit how much she could do as a mentor and weaken her freedom to act. The senior nurse mentor described in this book has responsibilities so all encompassing that in most cases she needs a full-time position. Larger hospitals may even have several. The military often aims for at least one person responsible for morale for roughly every 125 staff.

That said, a senior nurse mentor would still resemble a traditional nurse mentor, especially in that the "relationship is built on trust and is confidential." That's a key distinction between a senior nurse mentor and positions in administration. In the latter, almost every issue generates a paper trail. That stifles communication and makes nurses fearful. Issues that should be discussed aren't brought up.

There are still more differences. The nurse mentor helps nurses that are either new to nursing or new to a hospital. The senior nurse mentor I'm suggesting doesn't have those limitations. She serves either all of a hospital's nurses or a subset of them determined by shift or specialty. There's no formal assignment that expires after six months to a year. If you're a nurse at that hospital, you have a senior nurse mentor assigned. All you need do is consult her.

You can see why that relationship needs to be permanent by what I've already described. Problems can develop after a nurse has been at a hospital for several years. Transfers mean a nurse who is experienced in one area may suddenly find herself working in an area about which she knows little. That's what happened to me when I transferred from the highly specialized care on Hem-Onc nights to the broader and more chaotic care on teen days. Some questions that troubled me could have been answered in a few seconds by someone more experienced. Instead, I spent weeks muddling out answers on my own.

That's where a senior nurse mentor would be helpful, particularly one who makes a point of checking up on those who are newly transferred, asking them: "Is their anything about this new assignment that has you confused or worried?" Imagine a nurse who says that she's having trouble handling her start-of-shift medications. The senior nurse mentor could reply, "OK, I'll come by on Thursday morning. We'll find ways to make your work go smoother."

There's another reason why that nurse-mentor relationship needs to be permanent and universal. New technologies and treatments mean that every nurse regularly becomes new in some sense. Central lines illustrate that. On Hem-Onc the lines were such a major part of our care and had been adopted gradually enough that the regular nurses learned what they needed to know. That's how I learned. Our only failure lay in training those new nurses.

Elsewhere in the hospital though, central lines simply appeared without a formal introduction. For a time, they were rare enough that nurses could be excused if they saw them as yet another IV. They needed to be *taught* to treat them differently. But no teaching occurred. Instead, the hospital had mistake after mistake, and its plans to purchase new IV pumps were only a partial answer..

There's a technical term that applies here. It's called a "single point of failure." In a badly designed system, the failure of a single component can result in the failure of the entire system. That's bad.

A well-designed system has no single point of failure. For instance, by itself, commercial electrical power is a single point of failure. A tree falling across a power line could shut off all electricity to a hospital. Yes, some equipment has built-in batteries to provide power for a few hours, but that's not enough. The hospital needs generators to keep the lights on, the elevators running, and the heating or cooling working. When it comes to electrical power, a hospital can't tolerate a single point of failure. It must have backup generators.

Teaching nursing skills and maintaining morale are at least as important to a hospital as electrical power. There should be no single point of failure. Yes, it would have been better if every nurse were trained in central lines as a matter of course. But that wasn't happening while I was there. Nor is that surprising. Administrators typically build on their experience. They focus on avoiding old mistakes and may not notice new ones. Even when they see the need for change, those changes have to go through the proper procedures, meet budgetary demands, and result in new policies. That takes time.

That sluggishness was where our problem lay. Central lines were new and the hospital did eventually learn to handle them. But that slow learning curve could have been rectified in the short-term if one person, tasked with filling training gaps, could pick up on a problem and deal with it quickly on her own initiative.

Think back to what I've described. The first nurses I worked with did not make air embolism mistakes. They were experienced enough to double-check after every IV change. But when that second set of nurses arrived, problems quickly surfaced. They weren't checking carefully enough, probably because they felt overwhelmed.

A senior nurse mentor, seeing the first of those incident reports could have—on that very day—began to question staff about the cause. Since she was *not* part of any disciplinary action, nurses could be open and frank with her. She could discover the cause and come up with a speedy response.

Speed matters, especially with new technologies. There's no time for officials to notice a pattern, for a committee to meet, and for training money to be authorized. All those introduce delays.

In contrast, a senior nurse mentor's position is all the authority she needs to act. She is her own boss and could respond within hours. She could give the training that some nurses need in a single meeting, perhaps even by working alongside them. After all, working alongside an experienced nurse is how I learned to handle central lines safely.

A senior nurse mentor could also help hospitals with the 'almost disasters' I mentioned earlier. That's when something bad *almost* happens, but is caught at the last moment. Such events give advance warning of trouble to come and should *never* be ignored.

Unfortunately, an administrative system centered on fault-finding discourages nurses from reporting mistakes that they *almost* made. The confidentiality of talking with a senior nurse mentor could ensure that those almost disasters don't become real ones.

In short, a senior nurse mentor would be a marvelous asset to hospital. Much like that special executive position at Boeing, she could investigate an issue fully and freely with an open mind. She could discover what the problem is and suggest how it could be corrected.

20. Promoting an Ethos

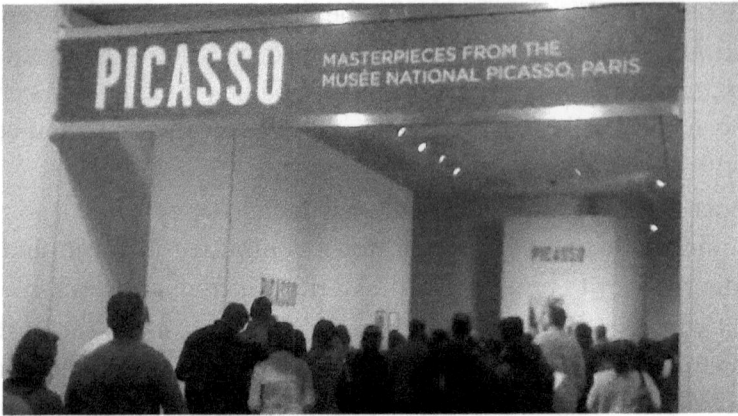

What should I do? I'd been told not to allow anyone but performers to park in the pavilion's underground garage. Some eighty were participating in a fund-raiser for Seattle's most prestigious art museum. They were performing for free, so the least we could offer was free parking. There were barely enough spaces for them.

Yet when I saw that elderly woman get out of her car and begin to hobble painfully toward the elevator, I decided to make an exception. Given her condition, I was *not* going to force her to park half a mile away. Most performers were young and healthy. One of them could park elsewhere. I rushed to offer her assistance.

About ten minutes later, the event's director came to thank me. There'd been a mix-up, he said. The woman was one of the museum's major donors and had been told she could park in our garage. What I'd done as a good deed proved good for the museum too.

In this book I've described several hospital situations when I did a similar good deed for our kids and was harshly criticized rather than thanked. Fortunately for those kids, I'm stubborn. I persevered even though I knew nastiness might follow.

The art museum was different. It encouraged those working for it to think beyond rules, policies and procedures. I wasn't aware that the woman was a major donor, but in the end that would not have mattered. I had a reason to make an exception for her. She was attending the event and needed to park in close. Flexibility like that was encouraged rather than punished.

I knew that because I'd been doing museum events on-call for several years. I liked the work because it fitted well with my writing. I wrote alone, so it was great to have a job that meant people. I had always considered myself an introvert, but to my surprise, I found I could easily manage a long line of people waiting to enter a special exhibition such as that for Picasso pictured at the start of this chapter. Some 400,000 people attended, and at times I felt like I had talked to at least half of them. Also, many events were in the evening when I was too tired to write anyway.

Working with the public goes badly if a set of rules intended for *most* situations gets rigidly applied to *every* situation. Airlines get in trouble making that mistake, as do public schools where a 'zero tolerance' policies often result in public relations disasters. Well-run organizations encourage flexibility and reward good sense.

An illustration of that came when I was checking tickets at the entrance to a exhibition of Roman art from the Louvre in Paris. A woman asked me if she could get in early because she had a flight out in just a few hours. Unfortunately, the general rules said I should say "No."

After she left, however, I recalled that she was wearing a badge for an event the museum was hosting that day for young professional women. Realizing my mistake, I found her and let her in early. Then I found all the others in the line who were attending that conference and quietly told them they could pass directly in.

That proved a good move. Just a few minutes later the talented director of the museum (and stepmother of Microsoft's Bill Gates) came to tell me that those women should be allowed in whatever time their ticket said. I told her I was already doing that.

I adjusted the rules on other occasions. The Louvre exhibition had a young Asian woman who kept coming up to the entrance to peek inside. Suspecting she was an exchange student who couldn't afford the $8 exhibition ticket price, I waved her in for free.

On another occasion, this time for the Picasso exhibition, I was managing the back of the line when a woman came with a problem. The exhibition was so popular that tickets sold after early afternoon had evening admission times. She'd driven many miles and not being admitted until evening meant she'd be getting back home late. She'd tried to persuade the less-experienced ticket checkers to let her in early and gotten nowhere.

That made no sense. It was late afternoon, the only time that hugely popular exhibition wasn't overcrowded. If she went in now, she wouldn't be adding to the crowding a couple of hours later. I told her how to bypass the usual ticket check.

Those examples and others illustrate why the museum liked me well enough to ask the agency I worked for to send me over again and again. I was so secure, I told people that if a problem developed with what I was letting them do, they could use my name. I did that because I knew that for the museum following its *ethos* was more important than sticking to the rules in every situation.

What is an ethos? Like any organization, the museum had "a characteristic spirit of a culture, era, or community as manifested in its beliefs and aspirations." **An ethos is the *why* and *how* behind an organization. An ethos justifies its existence and should shape all that it does.**

The most obvious examples of that museum's ethos were the first two incidents I described. Art museums, I learned, can't survive on mere ticket sales. They need large contributions from the well-to-do. To keep them generous, those people get special parking and skip lines. The badge those professional women were wearing said "VIP," museum-speak for "Give them what they want." That I did.

On another occasion I was working an exhibition's exit when the director came to tell us she'd be bringing a group of VIP guests through and that we weren't to hinder them. She was being careful. One of the exit staff saying, "I'm sorry, but you can't do that," would be embarrassing if the person spoken to was the museum's director. I knew her and would have let her lead in a herd of buffalo, but some of those I was working with didn't and might be sticklers for rules.

I should make an aside here. If you have a problem with that special treatment, keep something in mind. But for VIP donations, many art museums would not exist. You're paying perhaps $15 and having to wait in line. They're donating $1500 dollars or more and getting to bypass that line. You're getting the better deal, so enjoy it.

Letting that foreign exchange student in for free illustrates a different aspect of the museum's ethos. Its non-profit, charitable status meant that it had a responsibility, as one senior staff told me, to not only to provide art education but to provide it for free in some situations. Tour groups from schools, for instance, got in free.

When I helped that woman from out of town slip past those too-rigorous ticket checkers, I was also applying that ethos by engaging in good public relations. Getting treated well after her long drive meant she was more likely to visit again.

Now for a distinction that's a key factor in understanding the problems I've described. Did the children's hospital where I was working have a similar ethos? It certainly did and I knew it—to provide high-quality to any child irrespective of a parent's ability to pay. That was a far more worthy goal than that for any art museum.

Ah, but there was a critical difference. The museum was *extremely* effective at communicating its ethos to those who worked there and insisting that it be followed. I've already illustrated that. When I helped that elderly woman, one of its top staff came down to thank me. On other occasions, the director personally made sure that staff understood that donors and potential donors were to be well treated.

I was impressed. Its executives had a hands-on approach to their work, not hesitating to mix with staff at all levels. Working special exhibitions, I met the museum's European curator, someone so gifted she had acquired exhibitions that other museums only dreamed about. She didn't hide in a remote office. She checked on exhibits and staff. That's hands-on management. At the same time, our responsibility to treat all visitors courteously was stressed.

In short, the museum not only had a clear sense of its ethos, the leadership, from the director down, made sure those who worked there understood it and were rewarded for following it.

I have searched my memory, trying to come up with similar behavior by the hospital's administration. I've drawn a blank. Other than a brief mention about providing care to all children by an instructor during orientation, I can't recall a single situation where its leadership stressed the hospital's overarching ethos to staff.

In fact, the opposite was true. The leaders were not even moving about the hospital, much less communicating that ethos. Keep in mind that the distance wasn't great. The hospital's administrative offices on the second floor were as close to patient areas as the museum's offices on the fifth floor were to its exhibitions.

Working nights, I didn't notice that lack. Since I arrived at eleven in the evening and usually left a little after seven the next morning, I wasn't surprised at the absence of administrators. In fact, I enjoyed the illusion of being in charge of a giant hospital. At night Hem-Onc hierarchy had only three levels—resident, nurse, and me. Of the three, I was the most experienced. That felt good.

Days were different. The teen unit was perhaps the busiest in the hospital and the one that managed the widest array of illnesses. That may be why, when Britain's Queen Elizabeth visited the hospital, our unit was chosen for her to see. She visited us, and yet I can't recall a single visit by anyone of importance in the hospital during my ten months there—not one.

We had visitors a plenty. The place was a zoo. Specialists came and quickly went. Our residents stayed a bit longer since the details of care were usually in their hands. Lab techs and their kin were constantly rushing in and out. But at this zoo, one species was conspicuously lacking—anyone in the administration. The museum's leaders had gone out of their way to talk with staff and communicate its ethos. Their counterparts at the hospital doing nothing similar. That was the root of many ills.

Antagonism was, I suspect, one reason why they stayed away. In this book I've described the war between the administration and its nurses. Not only did many nurses feel under attack, the administration behaved as if it were under siege by an army of blundering, incompetent nurses. That killed communication.

One reason may have been the difference between what these administrators *thought* they would see on the hospital's floors with what they would *actually see*. They thought they'd see what some head nurses were telling them—poor nursing in need of stern discipline. As a result, they never saw real problems like those I described in my resignation letter—dedicated, capable but terribly overworked nurses.

Even less defensible were the two permanent head nurses who were at different times my immediate bosses. Each had offices at the entrance of their respective units, and yet they rarely moved about a unit only yards away. On the medical unit, when the head nurse arrived at six in the morning, she typically spent about ten minutes at the Hem-Onc nursing station before disappearing into her office. During my ten months on the teen unit, I don't recall a single occasion when I saw its head nurse moving about the unit, checking up on nurses and patients. Paperwork got more attention than staff work.

At the time, that seemed strange. Now I see it as one reason for the morale crisis. An administration seeing little and teaching nothing about the hospital's official ethos had by default brought into existence a different ethos, one of criticism and blame rather than cooperation and learning.

Fortunately, there were impromptu efforts to promote a more caring ethos by individual staff. On their own initiative nurses on one unit would let nurses on another unit know how a child transferred to them was doing. For Hem-Onc, that meant personal interaction with ICU nurses. Also, the picture at the start of Chapter 4 is from a birthday party held for a little boy with leukemia organized by a social worker and the nurse who dealt with family issues. Consciously or unconsciously, they wanted to stress that ethos.

In my frustration, I tried something similar about the same time. Without bothering to get permission, I posted pictures I had taken of our kids and nurses on the wall leading to Hem-Onc and offered prints at cost. I was saying, "These kids are what matters not these squabbles." The idea proved so popular that for many of those pictures the only copies I have today are the film negatives. Fortunately for me, the popularity of that idea made it impossible for the head nurse to do her usual ill-tempered squawking.

Alas, none of those efforts were enough to counter that distorted ethos. For that, a senior nurse mentor would have been helpful. In fact, one of her most important jobs is to constantly communicate a hospital's good ethos to its staff.

With the next chapter, I close this book.

21. THE TIME TO ACT

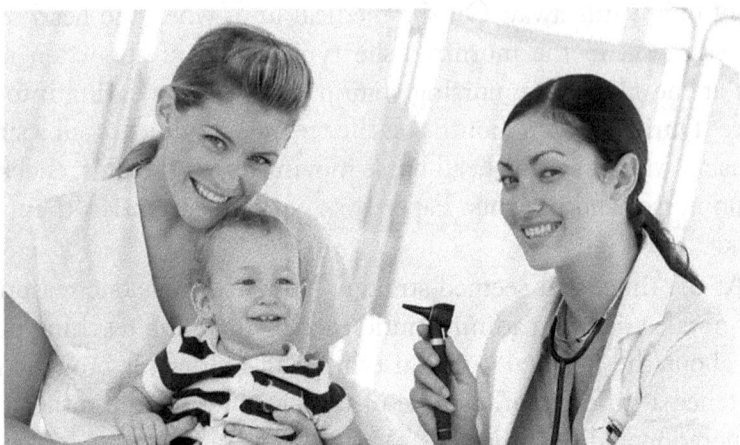

What's happening to this nurse?, I thought. Why is she acting crazy? Making matters worse, she was one of the two talented nurses in that second set of hires. For months we'd worked well together as a team. Now what she was doing made no sense.

We were on the medical unit's cluster most removed from Hem-Onc, the one we joked was for "poopers and croupers," since it had isolation rooms for children with infections. In one was a little two-year-old boy battling the flu. We normally took temperatures under an arm, but for him an anal thermometer had been ordered. I had done that and was leaving when she pounced.

Angrily, she asked me why I had waited in the room for the two minutes it took for a temperature reading when I could have done something else during that time.

Alas, I responded with equal heat. First, I told her, I never left a child with a glass thermometer in his backside—never. If he rolled over, it could have broken off inside him. Second, this kid might have pulled the thermometer out and hurled it onto the floor, where it could have broken, scattering glass and mercury around the room. Cleaning that up would be messy. Third, by the time I went through the isolation procedure both coming and going, I wouldn't have saved any time.

She stalked off, obviously unsatisfied. I returned to my work, wondering what was wrong. Her usual good sense had fled. Nothing like that had happened before.

About an hour later I noticed that she'd not done something she'd promised. Normally, I did all the vital signs. This night, she told me she'd do them for one of our isolation patients. Usually vital signs were done by midnight. It was now thirty minutes past and that child's weren't done. I was caught up, so I went in and did them. She was clearly under pressure. I thought I'd help.

Again, she pounced. Why had I done what she was going to do? This time I resisted the impulse to point out that she hadn't done the vital signs in a timely fashion and that, if she wanted, she could still go in and check on that patient. She stalked off. Once more, I wondered what had come over her.

Worse was yet to come. A few minutes later I left the side of a crib down, something that in her dour mood she was quite happy to point out to me. This time I didn't protest because she was right. I also began some serious thinking.

There was no danger for the boy in that crib. He was big enough that, if he'd decided to get down, he would have lowered himself to the floor safely. But I found my mistake disturbing. During my twenty-six months at that hospital I lowered the sides of cribs and the railings on beds many thousands of times. This was the only time, before or after, that I failed to raise one back up.

I realized what was happening. The ill-tempered day nurses rarely attacked me and when they did, I easily brushed off what they said. The head nurse's criticisms had a similar effect. What she said was so unfair, I concluded that, if her criticism had to be that contrived, I must be doing good work.

But the night nurses were different. Their opinions mattered and particularly that nurse. I hadn't built up any defenses against attacks from her, hence my reaction and the crib blunder that followed.

That clash did have one good result. I better understood why the nurses I worked with had trouble coping with attacks by day nurses and the head nurse. New to nursing and eager to please more experienced (or at least older) nurses, they didn't know how to react when attacked. The results were mistakes, some serious. Their very desire to be good nurses caused stresses that led to mistakes. That's bad, very bad.

Near the end of the shift, I discovered why the nurse I was working with had behaved so strangely. She told me that just after night shift she would face her first three-month evaluation. I couldn't see any reasonable cause for her to worry. She was a good nurse and becoming better every shift she worked. Unfortunately, she was too new to feel secure, and, given the growing hostility on our unit, she did have cause to fear an unfair critique. Harsh criticism was now the norm. I just wished she hadn't picked on me.

That clash bothered me immensely. I saw that the nastiness of those day nurses and the head nurse were now disrupting staff relationships *within* night shift and making it hard for me to carry out my responsibilities. That would play a major role in my decision to transfer.

As many of my readers are aware, my experience was not that unusual. Similar tensions arise thousands of times a day in hospitals across the country. That's not all. Research done over almost a quarter of a century by Dr. Judith Briles suggests that the situation is not only bad, it's growing worse. In her *Zapping Conflict in the Health Care Workplace* she writes: "The key factor in the nursing shortage is *not* that there aren't enough nurses. The key factor is that there is too much bullying, sabotage, undermining, and conflict in their workplaces." She is quite right.

The consequences of hostile work environments are disastrous. What was in my case merely a crib railing left down would, in just a few weeks, result in a night nurse so distraught that she unthinkingly followed an order for a ten-fold overdose of morphine that almost killed a two-year-old boy. *That* was when I knew I had to leave.

But notice that leaving was my only option. I knew of no one with whom I could discuss these growing tensions. The nurses I worked with were either the cause of the troubles (a few) or its victims (the majority). Our head nurse was worthless. I'd seen her demean staff repeatedly. Last but not least, the upper levels of the hospital's administration were too remote for me to approach easily, and their response was too uncertain.

I'll close by repeating this book's central message. Hospitals often develop a hostile work environment that destroys nursing morale, harms patient care, and results in a high turnover rate. The solution is a nursing specialty empowered to deal with those problems—a senior nurse mentor. Chosen wisely, she could transform the care-giving ethos of a hospital, making it better for all concerned—administration, staff and patients.

We can't afford to wait. The need is great. The future of nursing depends on us. The time to act is now.

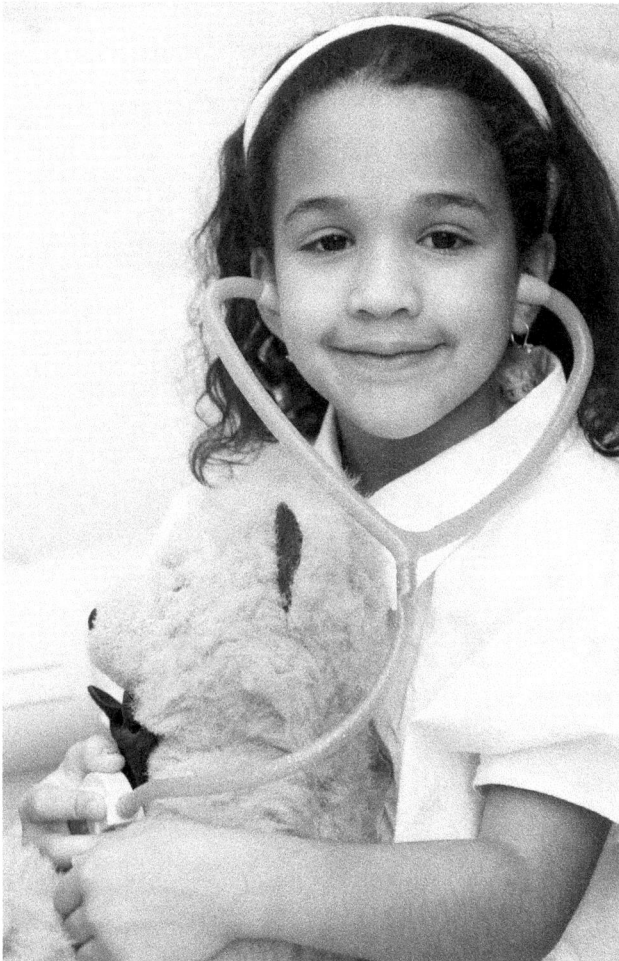

www.ingramcontent.com/pod-product-compliance
Lightning Source LLC
Chambersburg PA
CBHW070934210326
41520CB00021B/6931